Q SOLUTIONS:

Essential Resources for the Healthcare Quality Professional

SOLUTIONS

Essential Resources for the Healthcare Quality Professional

EDITORS

Luc R. Pelletier, MSN APRN BC CPHQ FNAHQ FAAN

Christy L. Beaudin, PhD LCSW CPHQ FNAHQ

NAHQ

National Association
for Healthcare Quality

National Association for Healthcare Quality
4700 West Lake Avenue
Glenview, IL 60025-1485
847/375-4720
Fax 877/218-7939
www.nahq.org

ISBN 0-9771100-0-1

Printed in the United States of America
10 9 8 7 6 5 4 3 2 1

For the National Association for Healthcare Quality
Executive Director: Diane K. Simmons, MPA CAE
Editorial Director: Barbara A. Simmons, ELS
Copyeditors: Juliette Kurtz, Larry A. Sawyer
Assistant Editor: Julie P. Cudden, MA
Graphic Designer: Robert M. Stoeck

Foreword

Founded in 1976, the National Association for Healthcare Quality (NAHQ) has as its goal the promotion of continuous quality improvement in healthcare through the development of professional expertise in the art and science of healthcare quality. Since then, the association has grown to more than 5,000 individual and 100 institutional members and is the nation's leading organization for healthcare quality professionals.

I consider it one of the highest honors of my association with NAHQ to be writing this foreword for a product we believe fully meets the mission and vision of the association. The product has been developed with feedback from the membership. It complements the other products NAHQ has developed over the years. NAHQ has always valued professional development, and this product is intended to enhance the skills of healthcare quality professionals by providing the resources necessary to carry out day-to-day activities.

I am very pleased to present *Q Solutions*. It is accompanied by a CD-ROM and a dedicated, searchable Web site comprising links to pertinent Web sites, measurement tools, case studies, and journal articles. *Q Solutions* provides in-depth information for healthcare quality professionals for developing and sustaining personal and professional growth. Very special thanks go to Editors Luc R. Pelletier and Christy L. Beaudin in their roles as team leaders—a Herculean, years-long effort developing this product. Thanks also are due to the authors of this innovative resource: Diane Brown, Jacqueline F. Byers, Jean A. Grube, Robert Rosati, Susan V. White, Danny van Leeuwen, and Lecia Albright. This team of dedicated thought leaders and experts has spent countless hours developing this multimedia product. An external review panel also provided critical feedback, and we thank them as well.

Q Solutions comprises four modules: Foundation, Techniques, and Tools; Strategy and Leadership; Continuous Readiness; and Change Management and Innovation. The resources and tools accompanying the theoretical underpinnings of healthcare quality are readily accessible. This product is a very useful tool in preparing for the examination to achieve status as a Certified Professional in Healthcare Quality.

As a purchaser of this product, you have been provided with a unique pass code for access to the *Q Solutions* Web site (www.q-solutions.org). Use of the Web site will be analyzed periodically to provide up-to-date content as needed. There also is a unique product evaluation survey site for providing feedback to NAHQ by completing a short questionnaire about *Q Solutions*. Data from this survey will facilitate evaluation of the product's effectiveness and inform improvements over time. The attempt here is to ensure that the product stays relevant to the ever-changing healthcare quality arena.

I congratulate you on your purchase; your decision is a wise one. I commend you for your personal commitment to professional development as healthcare quality professionals. In turn, we trust that you will continuously deploy NAHQ's vision: Healthcare quality for everyone.

John Hartley, MS BS CPHQ FNAHQ
2004–2005 NAHQ President

Contents

Module One: Foundation, Techniques, and Tools

Jacqueline Fowler Byers, PhD RN CPHQ CNAA, and Robert J. Rosati, PhD

Module One (continued)

Module Two: Strategy and Leadership

Jean Grube, PhD MBA MSN

Module Three (continued)

Module Four: Change Management and Innovation

Susan V. White, PhD RN CPHQ FNAHQ

List of Tables

List of Figures

List of Figures (continued)

Preface

Developing and deploying appropriate strategies is a continual challenge for leaders in healthcare quality. Strategies must employ effective and efficient tactics for measuring, monitoring, and determining actions and interventions that produce sustainable or improved healthcare quality. Healthcare is complex. Delivery systems, health plans, solo and group practitioners, employers, and government agencies seek ways to ensure quality while controlling costs. The healthcare quality professional must successfully navigate the system to demonstrate quality. The application of sound theoretical and methodological practices is imperative. *Q Solutions* covers the breadth and depth of the areas critical to professional development and leadership: frameworks for quality management, linking of science with practice, and the translation of data into information that can be used and understood by any customer, be it practitioner, purchaser, or consumer.

Since 1986 the National Association for Healthcare Quality (NAHQ) and the Healthcare Quality Certification Board have used the *NAHQ Guide to Quality Management* (the 8th edition was published in 1998) as the seminal source document for healthcare quality professionals seeking certification. Now *Q Solutions* moves beyond that foundation. Key features highlight critical components of healthcare quality, the science and art of quality management, and environmental and sphere-of-influence considerations. The work of healthcare quality professionals is noble indeed. Armed with a set of advanced skills and practical tools, we are a force that can be boundless. Our nobleness comes from the fact that we are truth seekers. We are constantly challenged to tell a quality story that is cogent and accurately depicts healthcare circumstances. To be able to tell the truth, we must demand the following from the organizations we serve:

- Provide resources necessary to conduct investigations and to maintain reporting systems that use state-of-the-art information technologies.
- Allow and support a solid infrastructure for continuous readiness, including health information technology, that supports the continuous quality improvement paradigm (and that doesn't disappear after an accreditation or regulatory survey).
- Ensure that appropriate staff are educated on the science of discovery (data, methods, analysis).
- Contribute to the growing body of healthcare quality science that shows evidence of quality techniques making a difference in the care and service that forward-thinking, high-performance organizations embrace.

And in our world of teeming technology, rapid innovation, and a continuous growth of science, we also rely on hope—hope that politics will not blur the needs of our customers and that resources will be available for the work to be done, day in and day out. And hope that fear will not result in resistance to uncovering mistakes, flaws, and failures. For healthcare quality to permeate the healthcare landscape, the cultures of silence that still exist in institutions that believe that their "dirty laundry" need not be hung outside for everyone to see must be identified and eradicated.

In addition to emerging technologies and techniques, the foundation of our work involves the collaborative relationships we form and develop with various stakeholders. Our work after all is relationship-based. Mutual respect and accord lead to mutual understanding and a sense of camaraderie as we face complex healthcare quality challenges. *Q Solutions* was developed using feedback from healthcare quality professionals and academic and policy experts in the field.

NAHQ's commitment to this multimedia product is to deliver healthcare quality resources in a variety of formats in step with current and anticipated demands.

Q Solutions serves as a primary resource for the rapid and continuous delivery of focused resources in a variety of user-friendly formats. It delivers current, anticipatory, and sustainable content to support healthcare quality competencies using the latest technology; is targeted to an audience across the care continuum; and provides critical knowledge to develop and enhance essential leadership skills in healthcare quality. *Q Solutions* core characteristics include the following:

- *Reliable and valid*—The information disseminated and exchanged via *Q Solutions* is timely, current, reliable, and valid. Customers come to rely on the information they receive from *Q Solutions*.
- *Sustainable*—*Q Solutions* is sustainable over time, and NAHQ ensures this by allocating ongoing resources to the project.
- *Innovative*—*Q Solutions* is delivered in various user-friendly and user-defined formats to reach the largest audience. NAHQ ensures that all members/customers have access to the content. Distribution channels are flexible, leverage technology, and change as emerging technologies are adopted.
- *Timely information/resource exchange*—*Q Solutions* offers timely dissemination of content useful to customers and employs continuous feedback to inform the development and refinement of content.

The writing of a book is an amazing journey. When we embarked on this journey, there was no question about who the right people were to make this publication "happen." We were humbled by the company we kept, and fortunately, these individuals made time for what has proven to be a fruitful endeavor. The product you hold in your hands could not have been possible without the unceasing efforts of Diane S. Brown, Jacqueline F. Byers, Jean A. Grube, Robert Rosati, Susan V. White, Danny van Leeuwen, and Lecia Albright. Their vision for NAHQ is depicted on every page. We thank them all for their thoughts and ideas throughout the development process. In addition, we appreciate the thorough content examination by our external review panel members: Suzanne Alford, Jon D. Beaty, Thomas Smith, Paul L. Green, and Bernard J. Horak. Many thanks also to the production staff under the thoughtful guidance of Barbara Simmons. And, as always, we acknowledge the continuous support of the NAHQ Board of Directors, which has resulted in the successful 21st-century launch of *Q Solutions*.

Editors

Luc R. Pelletier, MSN APRN BC CPHQ FNAHQ FAAN
San Diego, CA

Christy L. Beaudin, PhD LCSW CPHQ FNAHQ
Van Nuys, CA

About the Editors

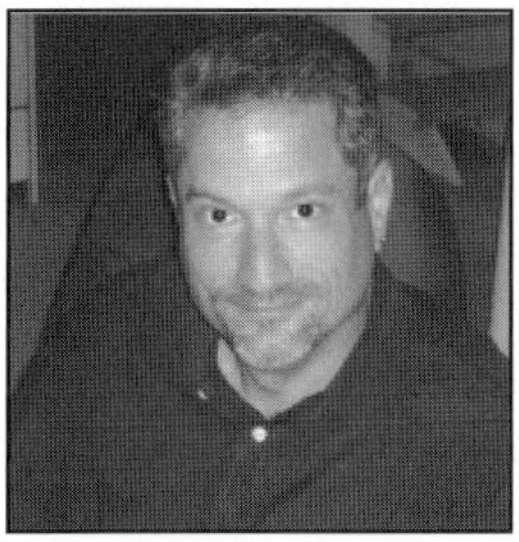

Luc R. Pelletier, MSN APRN BC CPHQ FNAHQ FAAN, is a healthcare consultant and project director at Danya International, Inc. He currently manages a Phase II Small Business Innovation Research (SBIR) grant, funded by the National Institute on Drug Abuse, Performance Measurement for Treatment Improvement (PMTI). The 2-year PMTI project has as its goal the development of a Web-based comprehensive performance measurement system. He is appointed to the faculties of The George Washington University, Washington, DC, and California State University in Dominguez Hills, CA. More than 20 years ago and prior to the current emphasis, Mr. Pelletier initiated the development of behavioral healthcare quality and performance improvement (QPI) standards. His integration of behavioral healthcare with QPI and publishing expertise has ensured the promotion of evidence-based standards, the consistent use of QPI approaches, and dissemination of scholarly work. Mr. Pelletier received an MSN from Yale University and BSN from Fairfield University. He has written/edited two books prior to this one, eight chapters in books, and 25 peer-reviewed articles, and published more than 45 other works. He has delivered presentations on various nursing and healthcare quality topics and given writing seminars to aspiring editors-to-be. As Editor in Chief of the *Journal for Healthcare Quality* since 1998, he coordinates the efforts of more than 50 editors, editorial board members, and review panel members. He is a Fellow of the American Academy of Nursing, the American College of Mental Health Administration, and the National Association for Healthcare Quality.

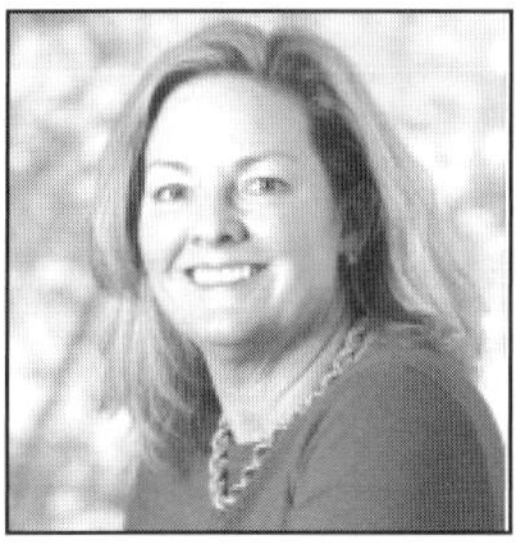

Christy L. Beaudin, PhD LCSW CPHQ FNAHQ, is Corporate Director, Quality Improvement, at PacifiCare Behavioral Health in Van Nuys, CA. She has more than 15 years' experience as a healthcare quality professional, having served at the vice-president level with other behavioral healthcare organizations and worked extensively as a consultant, health services researcher, and clinician. She serves as a national subject matter expert on behavioral health and managed care. Dr. Beaudin has supported healthcare organizations with preparation for and maintenance of state licensure and NCQA, URAC, and JCAHO accreditation. Dr. Beaudin earned her doctorate in health services from the UCLA School of Public Health, master's degree in social work from San Diego State University, and bachelor's degree in Criminal Justice from California State University San Bernardino. She is a member of the *Journal for Healthcare Quality* Editorial Board. Dr. Beaudin' s appointments include the URAC Health Standards Committee and NCQA Technical Subgroups for preventive health and HEDIS measures.

About the Authors

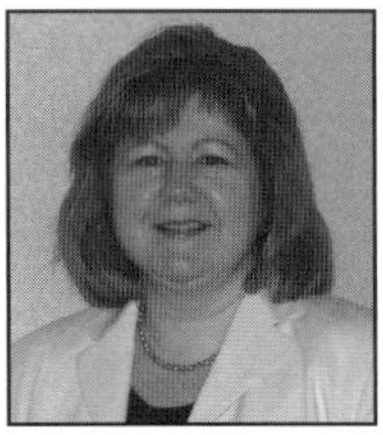

Lecia A. Albright, CPHQ, is the principal and owner of LARA Consulting, LLC, Fredericksburg, VA. Ms. Albright has 27 years' experience as a healthcare administrator and performance improvement (PI) consultant in healthcare organizations in Pennsylvania, Connecticut, Virginia, and Washington, DC. Throughout her career she has directed programs in hospital-based ambulatory care, emergency medicine, inpatient and outpatient rehabilitation, and geriatrics. In her quality improvement roles, Ms. Albright has acted as internal consultant and facilitator for the development and implementation of hospital-wide PI, and patient safety programs. She currently works as a consultant in her own firm, providing services to healthcare clients in the areas of accreditation survey readiness, PI, and patient safety. Ms. Albright is a board member of the Virginia Association for Healthcare Quality and its newsletter editor. She currently serves as *Journal for Healthcare Quality* Media Editor. Ms. Albright also serves as a mentor to healthcare administration students at the Pennsylvania State University's College of Health and Human Development's Women's Leadership Initiative.

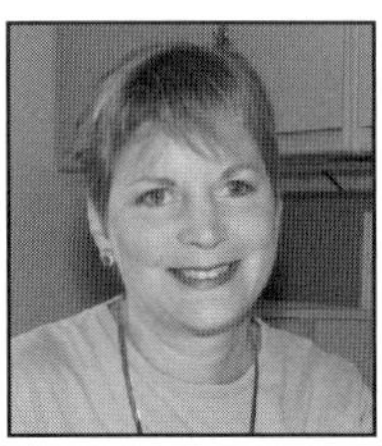

Jacqueline Fowler Byers, PhD RN CPHQ CNAA, is an Associate Professor, School of Nursing, College of Health and Public Affairs, at the University of Central Florida. She has more than 25 years of experience in healthcare in varied clinical, educational, and administrative roles. In all these roles, Dr. Byers has pursued evidence-based practice and improved patient experience and outcomes. She has been actively involved in quality management, outcomes research, and patient safety for 10 years. She received her doctorate from the University of Florida in 1996. Her master's degree is from Vanderbilt University and her bachelor's degree from Duke University. She was in the inaugural class of the Robert Wood Johnson Executive Nurse Fellowship program. Dr. Byers serves as *Journal for Healthcare Quality* Research Editor and as a peer reviewer for several journals. She is the co-author of *Patient Safety: Principles and Practice*, published in 2004 by Springer Publishing Company. She is active in the National Association for Healthcare Quality and the American Association of Critical Care Nurses. Dr. Byers has received a number of awards and has more than 60 publications and 100 presentations in the areas of healthcare administration, quality management, critical care, and outcomes and efficacy research to her credit.

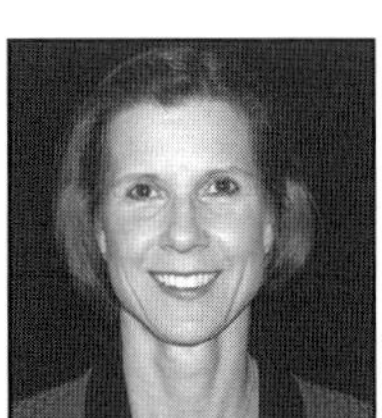

Diane Brown, PhD MSN RN CPHQ FNAHQ, is Director of Quality and Continuous Readiness for Accreditation, Regulation, and Licensing for the Kaiser Permanente Northern California Region. Her 25 years of professional experience include hospital nursing administration and university education roles in California and Oregon hospitals, including her current position at the University of California, San Francisco School of Nursing as an Assistant Clinical Professor, and critical care clinical nursing roles in Wisconsin, Nevada, Oregon, and California. Currently she is the co-principal investigator for the California Nursing Outcomes Coalition Project (CalNOC) and a co-investigator of several funded grants. She received her bachelor of science in nursing from Viterbo University in LaCrosse, WI, and her master's degree and PhD in nursing from the University of California, San Francisco. Dr. Brown has professional affiliations with the American Nurses Association (ANA), ANA/California, Association of California Nursing Leaders (ACNL), California Association for Healthcare Quality, and the National Association for Healthcare Quality. She is a member of Sigma Theta Tau (STT), serves on the *Journal for Healthcare Quality* Editorial Board, and is a manuscript reviewer for *Clinical Nursing Research Journal* and *Western Journal of Nursing Research*. She has received peer recognition from ACNL with the Excellence in Advancement of Clinical Practice Award and from STT with the Nursing Research Excellence Award.

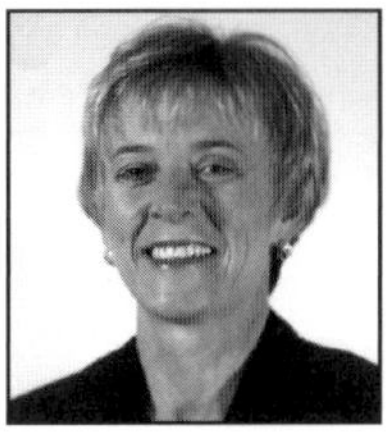

Jean A. Grube, PhD MBA MSN, is an Adjunct Assistant Professor in the Department of Family and Community Medicine and affiliate faculty in the Injury Research Center at the Medical College of Wisconsin, where she was formerly the Patient Safety Intervention Director on an AHRQ-funded Patient Safety Reporting Research Demonstration Project. She is also an Adjunct Assistant Professor in the Department of Healthcare Administration at Virginia Commonwealth University, where she teaches in the Executive Fellowship in Patient Safety Program and mentors fellows completing required patient safety projects. Dr. Grube is visiting faculty in the Department of Sociology at the University of Wisconsin–Madison, where she researches organizational behavior as it relates to quality outcomes. Dr. Grube also has publications and extensive experience as a consultant pertaining to quality improvement, employee turnover, absenteeism, leadership and management, and job satisfaction, and has served as principal investigator for a grant examining the influence of cultural values on organizational performance. Dr. Grube received a PhD in organizational behavior, an MBA in management, and a master's degree in critical care nursing from the University of Wisconsin–Madison. She is a past Editor and present Editorial Board member of the *Journal for Healthcare Quality* and is a peer reviewer for several other journals. She serves on the Advisory Board for Wisconsin's Quality Improvement Organization (QIO) Nursing Home Quality Indicator Project commissioned by the Centers for Medicare & Medicaid Services.

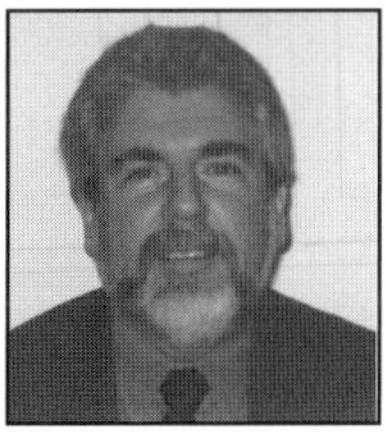

Robert J. Rosati, PhD, is Director of Outcomes Analysis and Research at the Center for Home Care Policy and Research, Visiting Nurse Service of New York (VNSNY). At the center, he is responsible for directing analysis and reporting of clinical outcomes for patients served by the VNSNY. He is currently on the faculty of Hofstra University, where he teaches courses in statistics and research design. Previously, he was the Director of Quality Management Systems for the Brooklyn Hospital Center. He also chaired the VHA Metro New York Clinical Improvement Steering Committee, which was evaluating care provided to patients in the New York metropolitan area. Dr. Rosati has more than 15 years' experience in healthcare in various research, quality management, educational, and administrative roles. He received his doctorate in applied research and evaluation in psychology from Hofstra University. He is a Contributing Editor of the *Journal for Healthcare Quality*. Dr. Rosati has published more than 20 healthcare-quality-related articles and made numerous presentations at national meetings. Dr. Rosati is currently a co-investigator on several AHRQ-funded studies: Working Conditions and Adverse Events in Home Healthcare, Patient Safety in Home Care, and Improving Transitions and Outcomes for Heart Failure Patients Through a Hospital-Home Care Information Exchange.

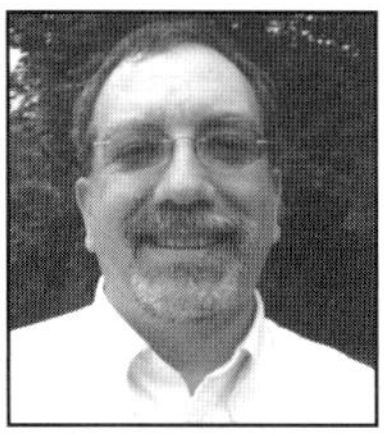

Daniel H. van Leeuwen, MPH RN CPHQ CHE, is currently Director of Professional and Community Standards for St. Peter's Addiction Recovery Center, Guilderland, NY, an integrated addiction treatment system and managed behavioral healthcare organization (MBHO). Previously, he was Director of Performance Improvement at Bassett Healthcare, Director of Quality Improvement for ValueOptions, an MBHO, and a consultant with the Healthcare Association of New York State. Mr. van Leeuwen serves as a leader in the Northeast New York Practice Research Collaborative. His 30-year career includes experience as a nurse, healthcare executive, and researcher. He has worked clinically in a psychiatric and a physical rehabilitation facility, in intensive care and emergency departments, as a paramedic in the field, and in homecare-based rehabilitation. He has attained national recognition for his published works in the *Joint Commission Journal for Healthcare Quality* and the *Journal for Healthcare Quality*, where he is a Co-Editor of the Quality Network column.

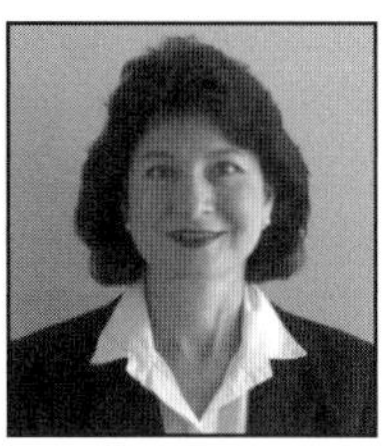

Susan V. White, PhD RN CPHQ FNAHQ, is Associate Chief of Nursing/Quality Improvement at the James A. Haley Veterans' Hospital, Tampa, FL. She teaches part time at the University of Phoenix Florida Campus in Orlando. Previously she was Vice President/Quality Management of the Florida Hospital Association. Her more than 20 years in healthcare includes experience as Associate Executive Director and Director of Nursing in a community hospital, where she developed the quality management program for a hospital within a large network. Dr. White received her master's degree in nursing, as well as her doctorate, from the University of Florida. Dr. White is a member of the Florida Sterling Council and has been an examiner for 6 years. She is a member of multiple professional organizations including the Florida Association for Healthcare Quality, Florida Nurses Association, American Nurses Association, Florida Organization of Nurse Executives, American Organization of Nurse Executives, and Sigma Theta Tau. She is a member of the *Journal for Healthcare Quality* Editorial Board. She has published more than 36 articles or books, including *Patient Safety: Principles and Practice* (co-author), released in 2004 by Springer Publishing Company. She has presented more than 36 in-service or education programs for her peers. She has certifications in critical care nursing, nursing administration, and healthcare quality. Dr. White is also a past member of the Accreditation Process Improvement Task Force and the Standards Review Task Force of the Joint Commission on Accreditation of Healthcare Organizations.

External Review Board

This project could not have been completed without the feedback from expert thought leaders in the healthcare quality industry. The external review board included representation from the NAHQ Board, *Journal for Healthcare Quality* Team, an academic setting, a member at-large, and the Healthcare Quality Certification Board. We thank them for lending their expertise in this process.

Suzanne Alford, BS RNC MPH CPHQ
Coop Retirement Services of America
Memphis, TN

Jon D. Beaty, LCSW CPHQ
Manager, Quality Improvement
PacifiCare Behavioral Health
Hillsboro, OR

Paul L. Green, MS RN CPHQ
Principal
Greenlight Healthcare Consulting
Palm Springs, CA

Bernard J. Horak, PhD FACHE CPHQ
Professor
Georgetown University
Washington, DC

Thomas M. Smith, MA RN CPHQ
Director of Medical Management
Health Management Corporation
Richmond, VA

MODULE ONE

Foundation, Techniques, and Tools

Jacqueline Fowler Byers, PhD RN CPHQ CNAA

Robert J. Rosati, PhD

I. Historical Perspective/Background/Current Initiatives
- A. Quality Management Philosophy
- B. Early Strategies of Managing for Quality
- C. Quality Management Pioneers
- D. Healthcare Quality Management Pioneers
- E. Current and Evolving Healthcare Quality Management Approaches
- F. Focus on Patient Safety

II. Institute of Medicine (IOM) Priorities and Competencies
- A. Patient Safety and Harm
- B. Changing the Healthcare Delivery System
- C. Policy and Healthcare Quality

III. Quality Oversight
- A. Public Reporting
- B. Rewarding for Quality

IV. Confidentiality Principles/Privacy/Patients' Rights and Responsibilities
- A. Confidentiality
- B. Medical Peer Review
- C. Utilization Management
- D. Medical Records

V. Evidence-Based Quality Management
- A. The Quality Management Research Continuum
- B. Evidence-Based Practice

VI. Decision Support, Risk Adjustment, Data Interpretation, and Benchmarking
- A. Decision Support
- B. Risk Adjustment
- C. Analysis and Interpretation of Outcomes Data and Decision Support Tools
- D. Benchmarking

VII. Systematic Healthcare Quality
- A. Development of a Quality Information System
- B. Strategy for Interpretation and Utilization of Information

MODULE ONE

VIII. Management Information Systems

A. Purposes of Information Systems
B. Implementation of a Quality Management Information System
C. Federal HIT Initiatives

IX. Quality Improvement Study Design and Analysis

A. Getting Started on Quality Improvement Projects
B. Data and Data Management
C. Data Collection Plan
D. Basic Sampling Designs
E. Data Analysis
F. Statistical Analysis and Interpretation of Findings
G. Performance Improvement Tools

References

Suggested Reading

I. Historical Perspective/Background/Current Initiatives

A. Quality Management Philosophy

The Institute of Medicine (IOM) defines *healthcare quality* as the extent to which health services provided to individuals and patient populations improve desired health outcomes. The care should be based on the strongest clinical evidence and provided in a technically and culturally competent manner with good communication and shared decision making (Committee on Quality of Health Care in America [CQHCA], 2001). As described later in this module, total quality management and continuous quality improvement are two strategies for achieving healthcare quality.

Total quality is best defined as an attitude, an orientation that permeates an entire organization, and the way in which an organization performs its internal and external business. People accept individual responsibility for the quality of their work and obtain genuine commitment and active involvement from the organization's leadership. People who work in organizations dedicated to the concept of total quality constantly strive for excellence and continuous improvement in all that the organization does. Total quality integrates fundamental management techniques, existing improvement efforts, and technical tools utilizing a disciplined approach and focusing on continuous process improvement.

This definition of total quality is applicable to all settings of healthcare. Regardless of the regulatory and accreditation standards that an organization subscribes to, the principles of leadership remain as fundamental elements of the enterprise's strategic and quality planning. The leadership is the driving force in creating and supporting the way people think about what they do. Leadership establishes the basis for procedures and focuses on the customer's needs and satisfaction. The leadership role must be genuine and visible, with active participation in establishing, achieving, and rewarding the attainment of quality objectives.

B. Early Strategies of Managing for Quality*

The need for quality has always existed. However, the means for meeting that need—the processes of managing for quality—have undergone extensive and continuing change (Juran, 1977). Prior to the 20th century, managing for quality was based on some ancient principles that included the following:

- Product inspection by consumers, which is still widely used in today's global village marketplaces
- The craftsmanship concept, in which buyers rely on the skill and reputation of trained, experienced craftsmen. Some craftsmen develop reputations that extend far beyond their village boundaries; they are viewed as living national treasures.

As commerce expanded beyond village boundaries and with the growth of technology, additional methods and tools were invented to assist in managing for quality:

- specifications by sample
- quality warranties in sales contracts.

In large towns, the craftsmen organized into monopolistic guilds, which were generally strict in their enforcement of product quality. Their strategies included

- mandated specifications for input materials, processes, and finished goods
- audits of the performance of guild members
- export controls on finished goods.

The early approach to managing for quality in the United States followed the practice prevailing in those European countries that had colonized the North American continent. Apprentices learned a trade, qualified to become craftsmen, and in due course might become masters of their own shops.

The Industrial Revolution, which originated in Europe, created the factory system, which soon out-produced the small independent shops and made them largely obsolete. The craftsmen became factory workers, and the masters became factory foremen. Quality was managed as before, through the skills of the craftsmen, supplemented by departmental inspection or supervisory audits. When the Industrial Revolution spread to the United States, Americans again followed European practice. The Industrial Revolution also accelerated the growth of additional strategies, including

- written specifications for materials, processes, finished goods, and tests
- measurement, and the associated measuring instruments and testing laboratories
- standardization in many forms.

1. World War II and Its Impact†

During World War II, U.S. industry was faced with the added burden of producing enormous quantities of military products. A part of the war strategy was to shut down production of many civilian products, such as automobiles, household appliances, and entertainment products. A massive shortage of goods developed amid a huge buildup of purchasing power. It took the rest of that decade (the 1940s) for supply to catch up with demand. In the interim, the manufacturing companies gave top priority to meeting delivery dates, so that quality of products suffered. The practice of giving top priority to delivery dates persisted long after the shortages were over.

During World War II, there emerged a new strategy: "statistical quality control" (SQC). The War Production Board, in an effort to improve the quality of military goods, sponsored numerous training courses on the statistical techniques developed by the Bell System during the 1920s. (Interestingly, W.E. Deming, who became widely known during the 1980s, was one of the lecturers at some of the War Production Board courses.) Many attendees of the training courses became enthusiastic and organized the American Society for Quality Control (ASQC; now known as American Society for Quality [ASQ]). In its early years ASQ was strongly oriented toward SQC, thereby stimulating further enthusiasm for the method.

As it turned out, most of the SQC applications in the manufacturing companies were tool-oriented rather than results-oriented. As long as government contracts paid for everything, the companies could not lose. In due course the government contracts came to an end, and the SQC programs were reexamined from the standpoint of cost-effectiveness. Most of them failed the test, resulting in wholesale cutbacks.

2. The Japanese Quality Revolution and Its Impact†

After World War II, the Japanese embarked on a course of reaching national goals through trade rather than by military means. The major manufacturers,

† *Reprinted with the permission of the The Free Press, a division of Simon & Schuster, from* Juran on leadership for quality: An executive handbook, *by J.M.Juran. Copyright ©1989 by Juran Institute, Inc.*

which had been extensively involved in military production, were faced with converting to civilian products. A major obstacle to selling these products in international markets was a reputation for shoddy merchandise, created by the export of poor-quality goods prior to World War II.

To solve their quality problems, the Japanese undertook to learn how other countries managed for quality, sending teams abroad to visit foreign companies and study their approaches. They also invited foreign lecturers to Japan to conduct training courses for managers.

From these and other inputs, the Japanese devised some unprecedented strategies for creating a revolution in quality. Several of those strategies proved to be crucial:

- Upper managers personally took charge of leading the revolution.
- All levels and functions underwent training in managing for quality.
- Quality improvement was undertaken at a continuing, revolutionary pace.
- The work force was enlisted in quality improvement through *the quality circle (QC) concept*. Quality circles involve employee participation in decision making and problem solving to improve the quality of work.

In the early postwar period, the affected American companies logically considered competition from the Japanese to be based on price rather than on quality. Their response was to shift the manufacture of labor-intensive products to low-labor-cost areas, often offshore. As time went on, price competition declined while quality competition increased (Juran, 1981). During the 1960s and 1970s, numerous Japanese manufacturers greatly increased their share of the American market; a major reason was the superior quality of their products. Numerous industries were affected (e.g., consumer electronics, automobiles, steel, and machine tools).

U.S. companies generally failed to notice the trend, continuing to believe that competition from the Japanese was primarily price-based rather than quality-based. Some observers sounded warning signals: "The Japanese are headed for world quality leadership and will attain it in the next two decades because no one else is moving there at the same pace" (Juran, 1967). The alarm was sounded at the Conference of the European Organization for Quality Control in Stockholm in June 1966.

The most obvious effect of the Japanese quality revolution was the massive export of goods. The impact on the United States was considerable, especially in sensitive areas such as manufacturing, steel, and electronics. The affected manufacturing companies were damaged by the resulting loss of sales. The work force and their unions were damaged by the resulting "export of jobs." The national economy was damaged by the resulting unfavorable trade balance.

C. Quality Management Pioneers

Certain important figures in the quality improvement movement viewed *process* as a sequence of activities and communications that accomplished a service for a client or customer (Gaucher & Coffey, 1991). The focus is on improving the process to improve the quality of the outcome.

1. Shewhart

In the 1920s, Walter Shewhart, a statistician at Bell Telephone Laboratories, developed the Shewhart cycle, known as Plan, Do, Check, Act (PDCA). This four-step process is designed to continuously improve quality (see **Figure 1-1**).

Plan. Question the capacity or capability of a process. Pose theories on how to improve the process and predict measurable outcomes.
Do. Make changes on an experimental, pilot basis.
Check. Measure outcomes compared to predicted outcomes.
Act. Implement the changes on a broad scale (Gaucher & Coffey, 1991).

The PDCA cycle was later adapted by Deming as the Plan, Do, Study, Act (PDSA) cycle; therefore, it also is referred to as the Deming Cycle, or the Deming Wheel.

Figure 1-1. The Traditional PDCA Model

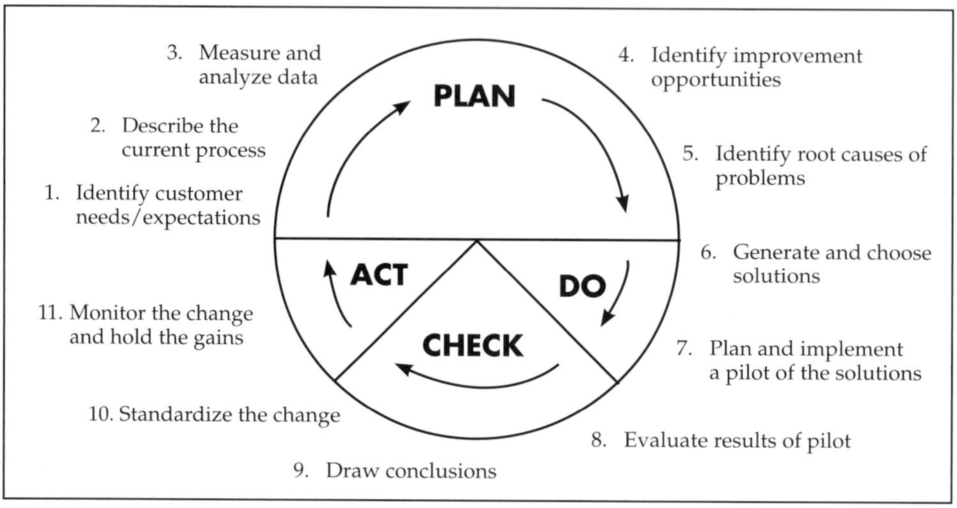

2. Deming

W. Edwards Deming is probably the most famous of the industrial quality "gurus." A statistician with doctorates in mathematics and physics, he ultimately became the "philosopher" of quality and the learning organization. The story of post-World War II America's rejection of Deming's quality exhortations—and of his subsequent dealings with a receptive Japan—is now legend (Merry, 1992). In the 1950s Deming had visited the Western Electric Hawthorne Plant in Chicago (while the Harvard University study regarding motivation of workers was in progress). Following this experience he proposed replacing traditional management techniques with a statistically controlled management process to determine when to—and when not to—intervene in a process. Statistical process control (SPC) techniques allow management to determine a range of random variation that always occurs in a process. SPC describes two types of causes of random variation: common cause and special cause. Common cause problems are rooted in basic processes and systems. Special cause problems stem from isolated occurrences that are outside the system. Deming said that 85% of the problems detected are process- or system-related, whereas 15% are traceable to individuals; this is known as the "85/15 theory" (Deming, 1986). Deming's management philosophy is based on his 14 points for business to be competitive:

1. Create a constancy of purpose toward quality improvement.
2. Adopt a philosophy that expects good products and services.
3. Cease dependence on mass inspection and build quality into the product or service.
4. Do not award business solely on price tag.
5. Improve constantly the system of production and service.

6. Institute on-the-job training.
7. Institute leadership with an arm to help people and machines do better jobs.
8. Drive out fear.
9. Break down barriers between departments.
10. Eliminate slogans, exhortations, and targets.
11. Eliminate number quotas and management by objective, and substitute leadership.
12. Remove barriers to pride of workmanship.
13. Institute education and self-improvement.
14. Take action to accomplish the transformation (Deming, 2000a, 2000b).

3. Juran

Joseph Juran's background was in engineering and law. He followed Deming to Japan after World War II, emphasizing the key role of top organizational leadership and the quality process in the organization (Merry, 1992). In the book *Juran on Leadership for Quality* (1989), Juran states that quality is "product performance that results in customer satisfaction; freedom from product deficiencies which avoid customer dissatisfaction." This concept is known as *fitness for use* and is explained in The Juran Trilogy®. Juran states that the cost of quality accounting means that there is a break-even point of less than 100%. Beyond a certain point, the cost of providing quality exceeds the value of the incremental improvement in quality. Juran's Trilogy is analogous to certain familiar financial processes. Quality planning is equal to budgeting, quality control (sometimes called *measurement*) is comparable to cost control, and quality improvement relates to cost reduction and margin improvement (Gaucher & Coffey, 1991).

4. Crosby

In the 1970s and 1980s, Philip B. Crosby developed an important concept known as *the cost of [poor] quality*. His work documented that high quality (what he terms "conformance to expectations") is actually less costly than the waste and rework that characterizes poor-quality processes. Crosby demonstrated conclusively that investment in quality can offer an enormous financial return (Merry, 1992). There are five stages of management maturity identified by Crosby in his book, *Quality Is Free* (1979):

1. Uncertainty, when an organization is characterized by the statement, "We don't know why we have quality problems."
2. Awakening
3. Enlightenment
4. Wisdom
5. Certainty, reserved for organizations in which top management proclaims, "We know why we don't have quality problems." The mature company is equipped to initiate a quality improvement program (Hunt, 1992).

Crosby identifies 14 steps to improve quality and to move the company toward "certainty":

1. Management committed to quality improvement.
2. Quality improvement team formed to oversee actions.
3. Quality measurement undertaken appropriate to the activities undergoing improvement.
4. Quality cost evaluated, using estimates as necessary.
5. Quality awareness promoted through various methods and supervisor involvement.

6. Corrective actions generated in response to Steps 3 and 4.
7. Zero-defects planning tailored to the company and its products.
8. Supervisory training undertaken at all management levels.
9. Zero-defects day held to celebrate a new performance standard.
10. Goals set for individuals and groups.
11. Error cause removed by management following notification.
12. Goals met and recognized.
13. Quality council's experiences, problems, and ideas shared.
14. Process repeated. (Quality improvement is a never-ending process.)

Crosby's underlying philosophy is, "Do it right the first time."

5. Ishikawa

Kaoru Ishikawa was one of Deming's early Japanese hosts and inventor of the cause-and-effect, or fishbone, diagram and is credited with using the term *total quality control* to imply not just the operational but also the total organizational commitment (marketing, finance, research) needed to fully actualize all components of the modern quality-committed organization. The preferred American term is *total quality management* (TQM; Merry, 1992).

D. Healthcare Quality Management Pioneers‡

A timeline for the quality movement, which began in the 19th century and continues into the 21st century, is shown below. The following sections describe these events in more detail.

Quality Movement Timeline

1863	Florence Nightingale calls for systematic review of patient care.
1910	Codman proposes end result system of hospital standardization.
1918	American College of Surgeons develops minimum standards for hospitals and conducts first survey.
1950	Donabedian formulates a theoretical framework for patient care evaluation (structure, process, outcomes). Joint Commission on Accreditation of Hospitals (now called the Joint Commission on Accreditation of Healthcare Organizations) is formed, accreditation of hospitals begins in 1953.
1960	Japan focuses on becoming a world quality leader, adopts Deming management philosophy.
1970	Juran and Crosby build on Shewhart and Deming's work; PDCA/PDSA cycles emerge.
1980	Berwick, Batalden, and James start applying quality improvement methods to healthcare.
1999	Institute of Medicine releases report, *To Err Is Human*.
2000	Six Sigma, Lean Enterprise, Rapid Cycle Improvements, Patient Safety, and Pay for Performance begin to have an impact on healthcare quality.

‡*Partially based on "The evolution of quality assurance and an overview of total quality management," in Merry, M.,* The Physician Leader's Guide, *1992, pages 28, 29, 32, and 33. Adapted with permission of Bader & Associates.*

1. The First Era: Nightingale, Codman, and the American College of Surgeons

Noting, in 1863, that patients seemed to fare better in some London hospitals than in others, Florence Nightingale was the first to call for systematic inquiry into the nature of care processes that might be related to this outcome variability. Although there is little evidence that Nightingale's quality vision came to fruition during her lifetime, Boston surgeon Ernest Codman's early-20th-century efforts had more direct impact. Also observing variability in patient outcomes among several hospitals, Codman called for a systematic evaluation process with a view toward improving care (Codman, 1916, 1972). Although his efforts met with considerable resistance, Codman's ideas were embodied in the founding of the American College of Surgeons in 1913. This body set about the task of establishing quality standards. In 1917, the college established a five-part "minimum standard," and the Hospital Standardization Program was born (Roberts, Redman, & Coate, 1987). The program was based on Codman's end result system of standardization in which hospitals would track every patient it treated long enough to determine whether the treatment was effective. When treatment was found to be ineffective, the hospital would attempt to determine why so that similar cases could be treated successfully in the future.

2. The Second Era: Donabedian, and the Joint Commission's Monitoring and Evaluation Process

Accreditation standards evolved slowly through the 1950s and early 1960s. At the academic level, the University of Michigan's Avedis Donabedian, MD, examined what research existed, formulating a theoretical framework for patient care evaluation (Donabedian, 1980). He is best recognized for his "structure, process, outcomes" model of quality evaluation.

This model suggests the importance of relating healthcare structures (the qualifications of practitioners and facilities/technology available to them) and processes (the activities involved in prevention, diagnosis, and treatment) to outcomes (how patients actually fare as a result of their care). In the past, Joint Commission on Accreditation of Healthcare Organizations standards mainly reflected the structure and process elements of this model. Surveyors reviewed the structures and processes. They assessed hospital plans and technology, qualifications of clinicians and administrators, and organizational structures against the annually updated requirements contained in the *Accreditation Manual for Hospitals*. Specialized standards for behavioral health and other services were developed as well. From documentation and discussion the surveyors inferred process. They reviewed minutes and interviewed clinical and administrative leaders to ascertain whether designated individuals were following proper quality evaluation processes.

As a matter of policy and practical considerations, accreditation standards did not address patient outcomes directly. First, there were problems with the way "quality" was measured. Second, no professional consensus existed on systematic measures of patient outcomes. Finally, uniform and comparable clinical databases were nonexistent. The problems of measuring and interpreting patient outcomes precluded their practical use in accreditation. As a consequence, the accreditation process was necessarily built on an implicit assumption that if proper structures and processes were in place, good outcomes were likely to follow.

3. The Third Era: Berwick, Batalden, and James "Discover" Deming, Juran, and "Japan, Inc."

The names of Donald Berwick, MD, Paul Batalden, MD, and Brent James, MD, stand out in the field of healthcare quality management. Like many of their colleagues, these physicians were dissatisfied with traditional healthcare quality assurance (QA) practices. These pioneering physicians, however, went beyond a mere critique of existing QA. Both Berwick and Batalden researched the industrial methods publicized by the Japanese experience. Arising from this research, Berwick's article describing healthcare QA as based upon the "Theory of the Bad Apples" has become a classic (Berwick, 1989). Among his many contributions, Batalden translated Deming's famous 14 points (Crosby, 1979) into a healthcare context (Batalden & Buchanan, 1989). In 1987, these two physicians played key roles in linking with the Juran Institute and a variety of industrial quality consultants to create the National Demonstration Project on Quality Improvement in Healthcare. This multiyear project and its original 21 forward-looking healthcare organizations conclusively demonstrated the applicability of TQM processes to healthcare (Berwick, Godfrey, & Roessner, 1990).

James, of the Intermountain Health System, was also a pioneer in applying quality improvement processes directly to patients and clinical outcomes. The success of James and his team has been measured not only in improved results in a single hospital, but also across the entire multihospital system (James, 1990). As more experience has been gained in applying TQM to healthcare, the list of visionary leaders, both clinical and managerial, continues to grow.

In 1991, Berwick established a not-for-profit organization, the Institute for Healthcare Improvement (IHI), which began driving improvements in healthcare by supporting national projects that focus on safety, effectiveness, patient-centeredness, timeliness, efficiency, and equity (the six primary areas identified in the 1999 Institute of Medicine [IOM] report; Committee on Quality of Health Care in America [CQHCA]/IOM, 2000). One approach was to set up collaboratives involving many organizations trying to affect the same issue and then use rapid cycle improvement efforts to implement change. A major benefit of this approach is that the collaborating organizations share their experiences and improvements spread quickly. Projects that have been initiated include improvements in chronic care, critical care, patient safety, and end-of-life care.

E. Current and Evolving Healthcare Quality Management Approaches

1. Six Sigma

In 1998 Mark Chassin, MD, concluded, "We can learn a good deal from industries that are working toward the Six Sigma goal. Let's try it in healthcare and see how close we can get" (Chassin, 1998, p. 587). Over the past several years, this approach has taken hold in a number of hospitals and health systems. With cost, quality, and regulatory pressures increasing within the healthcare industry, Six Sigma is drawing increased attention from hospitals and health systems seeking a better approach to achieving long-term results. The Six Sigma approach to improving quality can be used to address many of the challenges facing healthcare, including resource utilization, patient safety, appropriate use of technology, and increasing market share. The Six Sigma strategy (Harry & Schroeder, 2000) is remarkably similar to Juran's problem-solving strategy (Plsek & Omnias, 1989), which has been applied to healthcare (Pelletier, 2000; see **Table 1-1**).

Table 1-1. Comparison of Six Sigma Breakthrough Strategy and Juran's Problem-Solving Strategy

Six Sigma Breakthrough Strategy		Juran's Problem-Solving Strategy	
Stage	**Step [Objective]**	**Phase**	**Step**
Identification	Recognize Define [Identify key business issues]	Project Definition and Organization	1. List and prioritize problems 2. Define project and team
Characterization	Measure Analyze [Understand current performance levels]	Diagnostic Journey	3. Analyze symptoms 4. Formulate theory of causes 5. Test theories 6. Identify root causes
Optimization	Improve Control [Achieve breakthrough improvement]	Remedial Journey	7. Consider alternative solutions 8. Design solutions and controls 9. Address resistance to change 10. Implement solutions and controls
Institutionalization	Standardize Integrate [Transform how day-to-day business is conducted]	Holding the Gains	11. Check performance 12. Monitor control system

Six Sigma is a rigorous methodology that uses data and statistical analysis to measure and improve performance. Quality is improved by eliminating errors in production and service-related processes. Six Sigma is based on the concept of the normal distribution or curve and the belief that there is a point, six standard deviations from the mean, where there should be almost zero defects. Therefore, error rates should not exceed 3.4 defects per million opportunities (dpmo). Six Sigma can be thought of as obtaining the right measures (or metrics) of quality, using rigorous statistical methods, and having a philosophy that is customer-focused and data-driven. A Six Sigma project can address process redesign, a problem that needs to be solved, a change that needs to be instituted, or a process that needs to be monitored. Six Sigma projects are managed by "Black Belts," who oversee the project. Black Belts are members of the organization who have been extensively trained in Six Sigma methods. Black Belts also must be experienced in statistical analysis and interested in teaching others. Projects normally are carried out by "Green Belts" (organization members who are knowledgeable about Six Sigma methods but who have received less training). For major projects an organization will also assign a senior manager or executive to act as a sponsor. Barry, Murcko, and Brubaker (2002) suggest that 1% of the professional staff within an organization be trained at the Black Belt level and 4% or 5% be trained as Green Belts. Six Sigma has been successful in decreasing emergency room wait times, reducing medication errors, and eliminating duplicated tests (Barry, Murcko, & Brubaker, 2002).

2. Lean Enterprise

The Japanese automotive industry initiated the concept of *lean manufacturing*, whereby great importance is given to reducing waste and focusing on those activities that add value for the customer. *Lean enterprise* has in its roots the work of Deming, in trying to improve quality, but also includes a Japanese approach to business management. There has been growing interest in applying similar principles in service industry environments, including healthcare. Lean enterprise includes the application of value stream analysis, a tool for exposing waste, and root cause analysis, which is a method for pursuing perfection. Lean enterprise also includes the use of new technologies to facilitate more efficient practices. Jones and Womack (2003) describe the philosophy in their book, *Lean Thinking*.

The major focus in a lean enterprise is to eliminate waste in the following areas: production, waiting time, inappropriate processing, inventory, transporting, and defects (Jones & Womack, 2003; Martin, 2003). One of the major distinctions of the lean approach versus traditional quality improvement is its emphasis on investigating new ways of getting things done and making the changes in a short period of time. The basic idea is to identify new procedures that should be more effective than existing systems in eliminating waste. Quality improvement has typically used the incremental change model, but lean enterprise is more about total redesign. A key element of success is the commitment and involvement of workers in the change process. The typical project will include cross-functional teams that have been trained in lean enterprise principles and tools. It is probably better for an organization to implement lean methods before considering Six Sigma, because waste should be eliminated prior to fine-tuning the system to deliver excellence.

3. Reengineering

In the 1990s, reengineering was one of the major initiatives in hospitals. Most of these efforts were focused on work force redesign. There was typically a focus on restructuring systems and departments into more efficient processes. For example, hospitals experimented with creating new positions that combined work from several different areas. A focus on cross-functional capabilitiess led to the dissolution of departmental "silos." A "patient services associate" would deliver meals, clean patient rooms, stock supplies, and provide patient transportation. Many hospitals thought that reengineering would increase profit margins and create financial stability. The problem was that reengineering often became associated with downsizing and layoffs. When this happened, employee morale declined and productivity suffered. Because of these negative connotations, reengineering has fallen out of vogue and been replaced by other improvement models and initiatives. The more contemporary approach is to consider adopting the lean enterprise method to increase financial stability by eliminating waste.

4. Rapid Cycle Improvement

The IHI developed the "collaborative" approach, termed the "Breakthrough Series," to bring about rapid cycle improvements. Fundamental to the collaborative approach is the acceptance of a model and establishment of infrastructure through which collaborating organizations can identify and prioritize aims for improvement and gain access to methods, tools, and materials that will enable them to conduct sophisticated, evidence-based quality improvement activities that they could not conduct individually. The key elements of success are enlisting a broad range of "partners," utilizing evidence-based practice to improve quality of care, and developing toolkits that contain essential information and resources for change. At the core of the collaborative approach are PDCA cycles that build on incremental improvements. The real benefits to organizations that participate in the Breakthrough Series are that they can learn from other organizations' successes and failures. Another key principle to the IHI approach is the concept of *spread*. IHI has proposed that successful small-scale improvement efforts initially will affect an individual organization and spread later to the industry (i.e., other hospitals) and eventually to the entire healthcare system. The spread is fostered through learning sessions in which organizations share their experiences. The IHI approach also can be adapted to a single organization (the work begins in a few units or teams and then is spread to other units and, eventually, the entire organization).

F. Focus on Patient Safety

In the 21st century, eliminating medical errors has become the major push in most of the healthcare industry. Whether the focus is on medications or surgery, the goals are the same—to assure patients that they are being treated in an absolutely safe environment. There also is a regulatory component to patient safety, as identified in Joint Commission, federal, and state mandates for the reduction of medical errors. There are many proposed solutions to improving patient safety, from computerizing order entry systems to having patients indicate on their bodies, using markers, the area to be operated on. To increase patient safety, healthcare organizations need to conduct a thorough analysis of where and how patients are at risk for potential medical errors. White (2004) suggested that approaching patient safety within an organization requires a review in six key areas: structure, environment, equipment/technologies, processes, people, and leadership/culture.

Evaluating structure involves reviewing whether the general facilities are designed to promote safety, the right supplies are being ordered, and that policies/procedures address safety considerations. Factors related to the environment include an assessment of lighting, temperature, noise levels, surfaces, storage, and ergonomics. Reviewing equipment/technologies involves an examination of labels, instructions, and safety features to be sure that potential errors can be avoided when using various devices. Processes can lead to errors, and there is a need to assess whether redesign would improve safety by looking at some of the following factors: complexity, inconsistencies, time constraints, and the amount of human intervention (i.e., lack of automation).

Understanding the effect of people (i.e., staff) on patient safety is very complex and requires attention to many factors. For example, employee attitudes, motivation, health (physical and psychological), education, training, and cognitive functioning can have an impact upon the likelihood of a medical error. Further, there is a whole body of research that has explored how humans interact with machines and the potential for deadly accidents. The leadership and culture of an organization can drive safety issues when there is a willingness to allocate appropriate resources (e.g., staff, equipment), analyze processes, implement changes, support nonpunitive error-reporting, and promote evidence-based practice.

In summary, any improvement efforts focused on eliminating medical errors will require a detailed analysis of the care delivery process and the resources to bring about systematic change.

II. Institute of Medicine (IOM) Priorities and Competencies

A. Patient Safety and Harm

The IOM report, *To Err Is Human: Building a Safer Health System* (CQHCA, 2000), clearly caught the attention of providers, payers, and consumers by showing the direct relationship between quality of care and patient outcomes. Further, Becher and Chassin (2001) have pointed out that patients suffer harm because of three types of quality issues: underuse, overuse, and misuse. "Underuse" is when patients do not receive beneficial health services (e.g., 50% of heart attack victims fail to receive beta-blockers). "Overuse" would be when patients undergo treatment or procedures from which they do not benefit (e.g., 50% of X rays in back pain patients are unnecessary). "Misuse" is when patients receive appropriate medical services that are provided poorly, exposing them to added risk of preventable complications.

B. Changing the Healthcare Delivery System

The IOM report continued to highlight the problems in healthcare delivery and reported, "The American healthcare delivery system is in need of fundamental change" (CQHCA, 2001, p. 1). It stated that healthcare frequently harms and routinely fails to deliver its potential benefits. In addition, it concluded that care was not being provided using the best scientific knowledge. The IOM report suggested an agenda for "crossing the chasm" by changing the healthcare delivery system. The agenda includes the following components:

- All healthcare constituencies (e.g., purchasers, healthcare professionals, regulators, consumers) should commit to a national statement of purpose for the healthcare system that sets six aims for improvement that can raise the quality of care to unprecedented levels.
- Clinicians, patients, and healthcare organizations need to adopt a new set of principles to guide the redesign of care processes.
- The government, through the U.S. Department of Health and Human Services, must identify a set of priorities to focus initial efforts, provide resources to stimulate innovation, and initiate the change process.
- Healthcare organizations need to design and implement more effective support processes to make change in the delivery of care possible.
- An environment needs to be created that fosters and rewards improvement by creating an infrastructure to support evidence-based practice, facilitates the use of information technology, aligns payment incentives, and prepares the work force to better provide care to patients in the context of ever-expanding knowledge and rapid change.

As part of the agenda for change, the IOM's Committee on Quality of Health Care in America established aims for the 21st-century healthcare system. The committee proposed six improvement aims to address key dimensions of healthcare quality that were performing at far lower levels than they should be. They suggested that healthcare at a minimum should be

- *safe*—avoid injuries to patients from care that is intended to help them.
- *effective*—provide care based on scientific knowledge as to who will likely benefit, and restrain from providing care when it is not likely to benefit the patient.

- *patient-centered*—care should be respectful and responsive to patient preferences, needs, and values. Further, patient values should guide all clinical decisions.
- *timely*—wait times and harmful delays for those who receive and provide care should be eliminated.
- *efficient*—care should be provided in ways that avoid waste, including waste of equipment, supplies, ideas, and energy.
- *equitable*—care should not vary in quality because of patients' personal characteristics such as gender, ethnicity, geographic location, and socioeconomic status (CQHCA, 2001).

Now the challenge exists for organizations to successfully meet the six aims. This challenge translates into organizations establishing a new environment for care. At a minimum there will be a need to make a strong commitment to change, starting to apply evidence-based practice, more fully utilizing health information technology (HIT), developing effective multidisciplinary teams, and preparing the workforce. External factors, such as aligning payment with quality, also will need to change.

C. Policy and Healthcare Quality

In response to the IOM reports regarding patient safety and healthcare quality, many private and public national initiatives have been introduced to improve patient care quality across all disciplines and the continuum of care. In addition, federal and state legislation regarding healthcare quality is at the forefront of consumer and media attention. Not all of these proposed regulations, however, are in the best interest of patients or consumers.

Healthcare quality professionals have an obligation to stay abreast of pending legislation at the state and federal levels and to provide meaningful, data-driven feedback to legislators. Frequently, well-intended legislation is proposed by special interest groups, without a full understanding of the complexity or lack of effectiveness of its implementation at the point of care delivery. In its *Code of Conduct and Standards of Practice for Healthcare Quality Professionals*, the National Association for Healthcare Quality (NAHQ) proposes that healthcare quality professionals agree to uphold and promote the dignity of the profession and be committed to

- practicing the profession with honesty, integrity, and accountability
- maintaining the level of competency as outlined in the Standards of Practice for Healthcare Quality Professionals
- seeking the trust and confidence of all customers
- supporting the Standards of Practice for Healthcare Quality Professionals
- respecting all laws, and avoiding involvement in any false, fraudulent, or deceptive activity
- promoting the right of privacy for all individuals and protecting the maintenance of confidential information to the fullest extent permitted by law
- using expertise to inform employers or clients of possible positive and negative outcomes of management decisions in an effort to facilitate informed decision making
- giving credit for the work of others to whom it is due
- aiding the professional development and advancement of colleagues

- using the Certified Professional in Healthcare Quality (CPHQ) designation only after passing the written examination and adhering to standards established by the Healthcare Quality Certification Board (HQCB), and continuing to maintain those standards through the recertification process
- maintaining membership in professional organizations as a means of promoting quality and professional growth, avoiding the use of such membership for the sole purpose of solicitation of business or for personal financial gain (NAHQ, 2004).

III. Quality Oversight

A. Public Reporting

Over the past decade there has been a major shift in healthcare, with an emphasis toward public reporting of quality. One of the original releases of data to the public began in the late 1980s when the Health Care Financing Administration (HCFA; now the Centers for Medicare & Medicaid Services [CMS]) released case mix-adjusted mortality rates for hospitals throughout the country. Eventually these reports stopped because of hospitals' criticisms of the case mix adjustment methodology. In the early 1990s New York State began releasing mortality data on open-heart surgery patients by hospital and ranked hospitals according to how much they deviated from case mix-adjusted values. Hospitals were then labeled as providing either "good" or "poor" care. Those that had poor outcomes were encouraged to improve their care processes. Eventually, New York State released data on individual surgeons and other procedures such as angioplasty. Those reports are still available on the New York State Department of Health Web site (www.health.state.ny.us/statistics/or www.health.state.ny.us/nysdoh/healthinfo/cs.htm).

More recently there have been several national initiatives, both governmental and private, to report on a broader number of initiatives and to include the entire healthcare delivery system (i.e., continuum of care). There is now an emphasis on reporting not only outcome measures but also process measures. Examples of government-sponsored reporting include CMS efforts related to nursing homes (Nursing Home Compare), home healthcare agencies (Home Health Compare), dialysis facilities (Dialysis Facility Compare) and, soon, hospitals. Some of the private reporting groups include Health Grades (physicians, hospitals, nursing homes), the Leapfrog Group (hospitals including process measures), and the Joint Commission Quality Check (hospitals). All of these reporting systems are using basically the same approach, comparing healthcare providers to national benchmarks and providing a rating as to whether care meets specific standards. It should be noted that although not directly involved in reporting, the National Quality Forum (NQF) has as its mission the endorsement of consensus-based national standards for measurement and public reporting of healthcare performance data. NQF has been involved in setting standards for a broad range of healthcare issues. Many of these standards are being integrated into provider reports on patient outcomes required by the federal government (i.e., CMS). For example, hospitals will soon be required to publicly report on Joint Commission/CMS-developed, NQF-endorsed measures related to their treatment of patients with acute myocardial infarction, heart failure, and pneumonia.

B. Rewarding for Quality

The next step beyond reporting on quality is rewarding organizations for having excellent outcomes. One of the key principles behind the development of Leapfrog was to support value-based purchasing. Leapfrog's mission is to reward healthcare providers that provide excellent care. Further, it suggests that the rewards for superior healthcare value be based on four critical ingredients: reliable use of proven methods to assure patient safety, improved clinical information systems, routine use of modern quality improvement methods in managing and delivering care, and routine and active participation of consumers in healthcare decision making. Purchasers are directly encouraged to shift their resources to better providers, to educate their employees about the importance of comparing the performance of healthcare providers, and to assist them in using the measures to make informed healthcare choices.

The federal government also is exploring the benefit of "pay for performance." CMS is testing linking Medicare payments to hospitals directly to quality of care. In July 2003, CMS launched a 3-year pilot program with Premier Inc., a large, nationwide hospital alliance. The test will provide financial awards to hospitals that show high-quality performance in a number of acute care areas. The hospitals will use evidence-based clinical protocols to treat patients with five conditions: heart failure, coronary artery bypass graft, pneumonia, hip/knee replacements, and myocardial infarction. The hypothesis is that patients treated using these protocols will fare better, with fewer expensive complications, postoperative infections, surgical wounds, readmissions, and other problems that occur as a result of less-than-optimal care.

In the Premier pilot, CMS will calculate the performance of participating hospitals in treating these five conditions using established protocols. In total, there are 35 different measures that relate to the five clinical conditions. Hospitals that rank in the top 10% will receive a 2% bonus for those cases above the standard diagnosis-related group (DRG) payment. Hospitals that rank in the top 10% to 20% will receive a 1% bonus.

The pay for performance initiative is being extended to physician reimbursement. CMS has implemented the Doctors' Office Quality (DOQ) project, designed to develop and test a comprehensive, integrated approach to measuring the quality of care for chronic disease and preventive services in physician offices. The goals of the DOQ project are to provide information for informed decision making and to support adoption of quality improvement strategies by physicians. The project will measure clinical performance and patient experience. Ultimately, CMS hopes that the initiative will lead to new methods of service delivery, expanded coverage of new types of service, and new payment approaches. In summary, physicians will be directly rewarded for improving the health outcomes of their patients by using evidence-based practices.

In 2003, General Electric (GE), along with Ford, Proctor and Gamble, UPS and Verizon, started "Bridges to Excellence" (de Brantes, 2003). Using the framework established by the IOM and creating a crosscutting group of healthcare professionals from the provider, purchaser, and administrative sides, GE set out to develop programs that would encourage leaps—not baby steps—in quality. The programs' objective is straightforward: Achieve a certain level of performance and get a per-patient bonus. They work outside the current scope of provider compensation so that incentives are visibly and clearly linked to quality improvement. They also work across all purchasers regardless of their contractual or network arrangements with health plans—self-insured or fully insured, health maintenance organization, preferred provider organization, point of service or indemnity. Examples of pay-for-performance programs developed by GE include

- *Physician Office Link*—Physicians who demonstrate that they have adopted better systems and processes of care in their offices receive up to a $50-per-patient bonus every year for all patients who are covered by participating purchasers and plans. These better processes are focused on clinical information systems that have evidence-based decision guides, robust patient education and support, and appropriate care management for patients most at risk.
- *Diabetes Care Link*—Physicians who meet the performance measures defined in the existing Diabetes Physician Recognition Program (DPRP, a program developed by the American Diabetes Association and the National Committee for Quality Assurance), which includes good blood sugar, lipid, and blood pressure controls in patients, receive a $100-per-diabetic-patient bonus every year they meet the performance measures.

For the programs that measure patient outcomes (Diabetes Care Link) rather than systems (Physician Office Link), allowances are made for physicians who care for sicker patients, and incentives and rewards are deployed to patients who better manage their conditions. The latter includes deploying comprehensive tools to help patients become more engaged in their care, partnering with their physician. The goal is to align incentives of patients, physicians, and purchasers to focus their energy on achieving leaps in quality.

Third-party payers are also starting pay-for-performance initiatives. All the major payers (e.g., Blue Cross, Aetna, Cigna, United Healthcare) have begun testing some form of linking reimbursement to quality. For example, in California a group of health plans has taken the lead in pay for performance and is proposing that indicators (e.g., preventive care, disease management, patient satisfaction) based on the Health Plan Employer Data and Information Set (HEDIS®*; NCQA, 2005) be used to determine reimbursement. These payers have stated that they are strongly committed to value based purchasing and quantifiable results (www.iha.org).

Pay for performance is not without controversy. The Medical Group Management Association (MGMA) has voiced dissatisfaction with United Healthcare's incentives because the group believes that the performance measures were developed without physician input and that bonus payments are based on efficiency rather than on quality and patient safety (Versel, 2005). MGMA claims to represent 240,000 physician practices (www.mgma.com). The challenges in gaining widespread adoption of these programs by physicians are formidable and have been highlighted by a survey reported in the *New England Journal of Medicine* (Blendon et al., 2002). In it, physicians gave little weight to the implementation and adoption of systems that have been proven to reduce and prevent medical mistakes (e.g., computerized prescription order entry) and very little weight to public disclosure. These positions are diametrically opposed to those of consumers, to the position of purchasers, and indeed to the recommendations of the IOM.

**HEDIS® is a registered trademark of the National Committee for Quality Assurance.*

IV. Confidentiality Principles/Privacy/Patients' Rights and Responsibilities

A. Confidentiality

Organizations are required by federal and state statutes to maintain the security, integrity, and confidentiality of patients' personal data and other information. An organizational plan for information management should address the critical balance between data sharing and data confidentiality. Although timely, easy access to data and information is required, organizations must also ensure that data and information are safeguarded. The organization is responsible for protecting records against loss, defacement, tampering, and unauthorized use. Each organization must determine the level of security, integrity, and/or confidentiality for different categories of information. Access to each category of information must have a functioning mechanism designed to preserve the confidentiality of data and information identified as sensitive or requiring extraordinary means to protect patient privacy. The related Joint Commission standard is "RI.2.130: The organization respects the needs of patients for confidentiality, privacy, and security" (JCAHO, 2004). Other accreditation bodies have their own standards.

Healthcare organizations must keep confidential all information pertaining to medical peer review and the monitoring and evaluation of patient care. All records that can be identified by patient and/or provider should be kept secure and confidential so that the patient's and provider's privacy can be maintained. This includes the medical record (in any format, hard copy or electronic) and may also include reports, abstracts of data, and supplies. Effective information management security and confidentiality policies and procedures in a healthcare organization should contain the following elements:

- identification of individuals with access to information
- delineation of specific information as to which individuals have access
- requirements for individuals with access to information to keep that information confidential
- requirements for release of health information according to the Health Insurance Portability and Accountability Act (HIPAA) of 1996
- requirements for removal of medical records (the patient's medical record is the property of healthcare facility); medical records should be removed from the organization jurisdiction and in safekeeping only in accordance with a court order, subpoena, or statute
- policies for protection of personal health information (HIPAA, 2002)
- a policy for handling the root cause analysis (RCA) reporting requirement if the organization is Joint Commission accredited. (The Joint Commission has four options for sentinel event reporting, with the options ranging from mailing the information to the Joint Commission to requesting surveyors come to the healthcare organization to review the medical records and RCA [JCAHO, n.d.].)
- mechanisms for securing information against unauthorized intrusion, corruption, and damage.

Figure 1-2 lists the elements of protected health information (PHI) in the HIPAA regulations.

Figure 1-2. Health Insurance Portability and Accountability Act Protected Health Information (USCFR 164.514, 2002)

- Names.
- All geographic subdivisions smaller than a state, including street address, city, county, precinct, zip code, geocodes (in some instances, the first three numbers of a zip code may be collected).
- Birth dates, admission dates, discharge date, date of death, all ages over 89 unless aggregated to 90 or older. Year data only may be collected.
- Telephone and fax numbers.
- Electronic mail addresses, Web universal resource locators (URLs), and Internet protocol (IP) addresses/numbers.
- Medical record, health plan beneficiary and account numbers.
- Certificate/license numbers.
- Vehicle identification and license plate numbers.
- Device identifiers and serial numbers.
- Biometric identifiers, including finger and voice prints.
- Full-face photographic images and any comparable image.
- Any other unique identifying number, characteristic or code that could be used alone or in combination to identify the individual.

Examples of information management confidentiality and security methods include the following:

- Portions of medical records may be stored separately, for example, if the record contains information regarding certain types of psychiatric treatment. The complete medical record would have to be available as needed for medical care and follow-up, utilization review, and/or in quality and performance improvement activities.
- Organizations can restrict access to computer files or portions of computer files with the use of security codes or by restricting certain computer operations to specific terminals and/or individuals.
- An organization that relies on computerized information should have an adequate backup plan for each computer application and extensive security firewalls.

1. Release of Information

A written consent is required for an organization to release patient information to anyone outside the organization. A typical release of information form should have the following elements:

- patient name
- name of individual/organization requesting information
- reason for release of information
- anticipated use of information released
- exact material to be released, including reference to PHI
- time that the release of information is valid
- documentation that information is released only to the individual/organization named above
- signature and date of the patient or legal representative (as defined by policy/state law).

2. Authorized Release of Information

Information from medical records and studies may be released without written authorization from patients to individuals and/or groups who have need for the information. This is regulated by national and state statutes. These persons may include the

- governing body representatives
- organization director
- healthcare personnel involved in the care of the patient
- individuals responsible for quality improvement activities
- individuals in the health information management/medical record department.

B. Medical Peer Review

The nature of the data contained in a medical record is highly confidential. Policies and procedures clearly define who may have access to a medical record and under what circumstances in accordance with medical staff bylaws, hospital policy, and applicable laws and regulations. Due to the complexity of those issues, consultation from general counsel regarding national and state statutes is critical. Practitioner profiles can be maintained as a part of the credentials file or in a separate locked file. Most states have laws governing medical peer review and its activities. When applicable, files, their contents, and meeting minutes should be marked as "Confidential-Peer Review according to statute X." Otherwise, a simple "Confidential" stamp will suffice.

A mechanism also should be developed to track activity on each individual practitioner profile. A log or signout sheet attached to each file should contain the date of request, reason for request/review, name of person(s) reviewing, and any pertinent notes such as requests for copies of the contents. Policies and procedures define the circumstances under which copies of contents are made, such as individual physician request. In accordance with medical staff bylaws and rules and regulations, a mechanism for release of information with specification of contents to be disclosed should be developed. This mechanism is in response to evaluation of a practitioner's competence for appointment and reappointment to other healthcare institutions.

Minutes of quality improvement activities are usually protected under the medical peer review statutes. Therefore, maintenance of confidentiality of records extends beyond credentialing to the entire quality improvement program in the organization.

C. Utilization Management

There are numerous issues surrounding preservation of patient confidentiality within the utilization management function.

1. Internal Review

Policies and procedures should ensure confidentiality during the medical peer review process. These should be consistent with organizational policies and procedures (usually within the health information management/medical records department) and may include completion of a confidentiality statement signed by staff and practitioners involved in the peer review process.

Mechanisms also should be established to inform patients of the utilization management review policies and procedures. A common method to inform and obtain consent is to include a statement on the admission consent form and/or consent for treatment form used by the hospital.

2. External Review

Review by telephone is a legally risky aspect of external review for the hospital.

The utilization management program should have written policies governing how a telephone review is conducted. These policies should address such things as methods to verify caller identity, determination of who in the organization may provide information to utilization/care management entities, limits on the information provided, and HIPAA compliance. Of particular concern is provision of the reason for hospitalization, such as substance use/abuse, mental health, HIV/AIDS, and other PHI as identified by HIPAA. These policies must be communicated to the insurance company as part of the managed care contract review process.

On-site review by external agencies also requires development and communication of, and adherence to, policies and procedures. Areas to be covered include proper identification of the on-site reviewer (photo name badge), issuance of passes to enter patient care areas, notification of the utilization management program representative on arrival and departure, and what information can and cannot leave the premises. As with telephonic review, these protocols should be discussed with the third-party payer during the contract negotiations and incorporated into the contract. The issue of patient consent to allow review by the insurance company generally is covered in the terms of the contract for healthcare coverage. During hospital/provider negotiations, healthcare quality professionals should confirm that the process occurs.

D. Medical Records

Healthcare facilities and clinical staff who treat patients are required to maintain adequate medical records to serve as a basis for planning care and for communicating about patients' conditions and treatments with other healthcare providers. The medical record serves other purposes as well. For example, medical records are reviewed by administrative staff performing quality, utilization, and risk management functions and by physicians engaged in peer review. Outside organizations also use the medical record for matters relating to payment and accreditation. In malpractice cases, the medical record serves as the major source of evidence about the care the patient received. Information contained in medical records also is used in retrospective clinical research. If PHI is collected for research, privacy or institutional review board approval is needed.

Healthcare organizations should have a clear policy about who may have access to medical records, whether those records are written, computerized, or otherwise maintained. Policy statements also should make clear what, other than actual medical records, constitutes a portion of the record. For example, with the advent of and frequent use of videotaping of procedures or fetal heart monitoring strips, it is important to address (based on state law and legal advice) whether such things as videotapes are part of the medical record.

The legal basis for confidentiality derives from the physician-patient privilege, set forth by statute in almost all states. This is one of several relationships recognized as special by law. The preservation of confidentiality is viewed as essential to the maintenance of the relationship. The need for confidentiality in the physician-patient relationship gives rise to a legal privilege. This means that, absent a patient authorization or waiver or an overriding law or public policy, medical information about a patient is protected from the process known as *discovery*, through which parties to a lawsuit normally can compel disclosure of relevant evidence. In certain states, the physician-patient privilege is extended beyond physicians to protect the patient's relationship with other healthcare practitioners (e.g., psychologists, clinical social workers, advanced practice registered nurses).

1. Information Covered by Privilege

This information extends beyond oral communication between practitioner and patient to cover written entries in the patient's medical record, as well as X rays, cardiograph or fetal monitoring strips, laboratory results, and other information concerning a patient's condition that is kept by the individual provider or healthcare institution. Information that is privileged must satisfy the following conditions:

- It must have been communicated in the context of the physician-patient relationship.
- It must have been given with the expectation that it remain confidential.
- It must be necessary for the diagnosis and treatment of the patient.

2. Patients' Bill of Rights and Responsibilities

Although specific wording may vary by state, a patient has both rights and responsibilities. A summary of the federal version of the Patients' Bill of Rights and Responsibilities is shown in **Figure 1-3**. A recent change in this area is the inclusion of patients' responsibilities to actively participate in promoting health, decision making, and care.

Figure 1-3. Patients' Bill of Rights and Responsibilities

I. Information Disclosure
You have the right to receive accurate and easily understood information about your health plan, healthcare professionals, and healthcare facilities. If you speak another language, have a physical or mental disability, or just don't understand something, assistance will be provided so you can make informed healthcare decisions.

II. Choice of Providers and Plans
You have the right to a choice of healthcare providers that is sufficient to provide you with access to appropriate high-quality healthcare.

III. Access to Emergency Services
If you have severe pain, an injury, or sudden illness that convinces you that your health is in serious jeopardy, you have the right to receive screening and stabilization emergency services whenever and wherever needed, without prior authorization or financial penalty.

IV. Participation in Treatment Decisions
You have the right to know all your treatment options and to participate in decisions about your care. Parents, guardians, family members, or other individuals that you designate can represent you if you cannot make your own decisions.

V. Respect and Nondiscrimination
You have the right to considerate, respectful, and nondiscriminatory care from your doctors, health plan representatives, and other healthcare providers.

VI. Confidentiality of Health Information
You have the right to talk in confidence with healthcare providers and to have your healthcare information protected. You also have the right to review and copy your own medical record and request that your physician amend your record if it is not accurate, relevant, or complete.

VII. Complaints and Appeals
You have the right to a fair, fast, and objective review of any complaint you have against your health plan, doctors, hospitals or other healthcare personnel. This includes complaints about waiting times, operating hours, the conduct of healthcare personnel, and the adequacy of healthcare facilities.

Source: Retrieved from http://www.consumer.gov/qualityhealth/rights.htm

V. Evidence-Based Quality Management

A. The Quality Management Research Continuum

Quality improvement activities and research exist on a continuum of rigor, as seen in **Table 1-2**. Both are based on the scientific method and are used to better understand phenomena. The scientific approach is the most sophisticated method of acquiring knowledge. This approach involves inductive and deductive reasoning to define a process that self-evaluates, in an attempt to reach conclusions superior to those arrived at through reliance on tradition, authority, and experience. Integrating the "right pieces" of data and information into a research-based framework for the study of people was a contribution of the earliest pioneers in the field of healthcare quality.

Table 1-2. Research Process Versus Quality Improvement Process

Scientific Process/Research Process	Quality Improvement Process
Identify the information need(s) or ask the question to be investigated.	Identify the process improvement, survey the literature, and flowchart the process.
Define the variable(s) or the elements for which data are required.	Define the customers and problem.
Formulate a plan of study or hypotheses.	Formulate a plan.
Choose or design the research design and collection tools/instruments.	Choose one or a combination of basic or quality management and planning tools.
Collect the data.	Collect the data.
Analyze the data.	Analyze the data. Look for root causes.
Display the data.	Display the data.
Report the data and findings.	Report the data and findings.
Draw conclusions.	Draw conclusions.
Act upon recommendations deduced from the conclusions.	Act upon recommendations deduced from the conclusions.
Continue to monitor the process.	Continue to monitor the process.
Evaluate and communicate conclusions.	Evaluate and communicate conclusions.
	Hold the improvement.

The underlying assumptions of design, measurement, and interpretation are the same. Healthcare quality professionals should use the level of research rigor that best answers the specific performance improvement question. There needs to be a balance between rigor and practicality. (See Byers and Beaudin, 2002, in the Reference list.) Research studies and systematic reviews can be evaluated for usefulness to a practice setting using critical appraisal tools. These tools guide healthcare quality professionals through the research critique process, allowing effective evaluation and synthesis of research findings for use in performance improvement activities. More information on critical appraisal tools is available in the supplemental materials (Byers & Beaudin, 2001). In addition, the supplemental materials provide Web sites that facilitate searching for the evidence relating to a particular topic.

B. Evidence-Based Practice

Evidence-based medicine is the "conscientious, explicit and judicious use of current best evidence in making decisions about the care of individual patients" (Sackett, Rosenberg, Muir-Gray, Haynes, & Richardson, 1996, p. 71). As multiple disciplines are involved in healthcare delivery, however, the term *evidence-based practice* (EBP) is more appropriate than *evidence-based medicine* from a healthcare quality perspective. Clinicians should base their care not only on the experimental evidence, but also should consider experiential evidence, physiologic principles, patient and professional values, and system features in their decision making (Tonelli, 2001). This allows individualized application and diffusion of aggregate research evidence (Greenhalgh, 1999; Tonelli).

EBP promotes patient safety through the provision of effective and efficient healthcare, resulting in less variation in care and fewer unnecessary or non-therapeutic interventions (CQHCA, 2001). EBP and outcomes measurement are iterative; one facilitates the other (Deaton, 2001). EBP complements the principles of continuous quality improvement (CQI). Outcomes evaluation at the individual and aggregate level is an essential step in evaluating the impact of EBP.

Evidence-based quality management is based on two types of research: clinical research and health services research. Clinical research evaluates the impact of interventions on patient outcomes. Outcome measures may include clinical outcomes, functional outcomes, and patient satisfaction. This type of research assists healthcare quality professionals in determining clinical evidence-based best practices. Health services research evaluates the health system at the micro and macro levels. Results from this type of research guide healthcare quality professionals in improving work processes and systems of care.

To facilitate research-based practice, that is, to promote research utilization, healthcare quality professionals must collaborate with organizational leadership to promote a culture of excellence. Healthcare providers must be motivated to provide the best possible care and to use the best system processes based on the evidence in the research literature or from data obtained in their own organizations. A key strategy is to keep all discussions based on improving the patient's experience and outcomes, and keep personality conflicts out of the conversation based on previously established ground rules. Research utilization is a key aspect of the CQI process and critical to obtaining healthcare quality as defined by the IOM.

VI. Decision Support, Risk Adjustment, Data Interpretation, and Benchmarking

A. Decision Support

Performance outcomes measurement or decision support systems can provide a primary focus to determine the quality of healthcare services provided to consumers. By analyzing data and information generated by an effective performance outcomes measurement system, healthcare quality professionals will be able to help identify areas for improving quality and resources in their organizations. Other uses for outcomes systems include helping to identify how an organization measures up in relation to its competitors, identifying individual providers and practitioners who meet acceptable levels of quality, allowing providers to respond more rapidly to market changes, and paying for exceptional performance.

Organizations should use available decision support systems to develop an outcomes information management plan, which includes evaluating performance outcomes measurement systems. Outcomes are viewed in terms of various clinical topics, including mortality, complication rates, infection rates, Cesarean section (C-section) rates, and other clinical outcomes measurement categories. Categories might or might not reflect the resources (cost, charges, length of stay [LOS]), associated with a given outcome.

To analyze and interpret such outcomes data, healthcare quality professionals would start with the type of system. There are two types: chart-based and code-based. With chart-based systems, nursing or medical record analysts review the medical records of all discharged inpatients to capture and input diagnostic, procedural, and detailed clinical findings, such as laboratory results. This is done to identify severity- and risk-adjusted information from the time of the patient's admission and at different points throughout the hospitalization.

Code-based systems are based on retrospective administrative data, such as data in the Uniform Bill document 1992 (UB-92) or claims data. These systems include clinical information spanning the patient's entire stay but not identifying the specific timing of certain conditions. This additional type of information can be available in a chart-based system. There also are some very significant benefits to using a code-based system, including much lower costs. Another benefit of a code-based system is that is it more likely to contain a sample size sufficient to develop more reliable models and output, and to provide sufficient and meaningful groups for comparing data. Most states require hospitals to submit all payer data that are deemed public information. These data can be purchased by an interested organization and then analyzed and interpreted using statistical tools, in search of key variables that might predict the likelihood of a desired outcome.

Both chart-based and code-based systems allow healthcare providers to identify areas where outcomes are positive and where they are negative so that appropriate action can be taken. Both types of systems serve to focus users on areas of concern regarding outcomes performance. Cost savings occur because energy can be focused on analyzing and controlling deviations from the baseline.

B. Risk Adjustment

Risk adjustment is a technique used to take into account or to control the fact that different patients with the same diagnosis might, in fact, have additional conditions or characteristics that could affect how well they respond to treatment. Risk-increasing variables reflect that a patient has a high probability of dying. Analysis of outcomes data using statistical techniques can take into account and control for patients' characteristics or conditions that are clinically meaningful and also have demonstrated a statistical effect on the rates for each condition. This removes the bias effect that can result when practitioners primarily treat patients who are more likely to experience desirable outcomes, such as patients with fewer risk factors or co-occurring illnesses (morbidities).

Some outcomes measurement systems define the differences between *risk adjustment* and *severity*, whereas other systems use the terms interchangeably. However, there is a difference. Patients in a particular study population may respond with either a "yes" or "no" when asked if they have had certain outcomes; the outcomes variable in this case is binary. The probability of a "yes" answer is the risk of the outcome. Statistical methodologies to adjust for the risk are applied to the outcomes data to predict the patient-specific variables, such as certain diagnoses that are risk factors. The validity of each risk adjustment model is assessed on the basis of the choice of risk factors, including both potential risk factors as well as those actually included in the model; and through measures of how well the predictions match overall experience. This assessment includes overall indicators such as measures of patient subpopulations, including patients with more than one risk factor; and the concordance statistic, which shows, in percentages, how accurate the model is at predicting the outcome.

The yes-or-no nature of outcomes data means that outcomes can refer to clinical outcomes, such as inpatient C-section complication rates. Outcomes also can be defined by using LOS and charges or cost, such as when an LOS exceeds a certain number of days and results in a "yes" or "no" answer. When the categories are in two or more groups, a set of outcomes can be defined and the risk adjustment methodologies can be applied to the full set of outcomes at the same time.

There is an important distinction to be made between the statistical analysis of X binary and continuous data. Risk adjustment methodologies do not apply to dependent variables that are continuous, like cost or LOS. The answer could be any number on a continuum, not "yes" or "no." Severity adjustment methodologies are applied to the cost of LOS data to predict severity by using patient-specific variables, called *severity factors*. Frequently, the presence of additional diagnoses helps to define the severity of a group of patients within a DRG or on an individual patient level, or both. Both risk-adjusted and severity-adjusted data are extremely important outcomes system tools.

Using unadjusted or raw data means that all patients in the clinical topic category, regardless of their health status or the existence of varying clinical conditions, are included in the calculation of the rates. Both raw and risk-adjusted data can be made available on the same outcomes topic, because payers frequently use risk-adjusted data in their initial decision making.

Healthcare quality professionals also must be familiar with how their decision support databases handle statistical "outliers." Are all patients included, or are patients more than two standard deviations from the mean removed from data analysis? Most decision support databases have a consistent approach to patients who are outliers. It is critical during data comparisons to make sure that all data sources have managed patient outliers in a consistent fashion. For example, a hospital physician group was trying to compare their performance on resource utilization and LOS for community-acquired pneumonia. They had one patient on their service that was hospitalized for more than 100 days, as he was ventilator-dependent and did not have adequate resources to be placed in an extended care facility. This patient needed to be removed from the data before a fair comparison could be made.

Another factor to consider in the analysis and interpretation of outcomes data is the level of detail. The best system is one that includes every payer's, every practitioner's, and every patient's clinical and financial information. This integrated data repository can mine data for

- benchmarking quality performance against established standards
- comparing physician performance within given outcome topics
- examining details at the patient level
- viewing patients' diagnoses, procedures, and other information
- determining the impact of managed care on costs and outcomes
- analyzing product lines to evaluate their effectiveness and to increase or downsize service offerings.

C. Analysis and Interpretation of Outcomes Data and Decision Support Tools

Healthcare quality managers facilitate analysis and interpretation of outcomes and decision support data for the organization. The reference point for the outcomes data must always be kept in mind whenever the results of such data are analyzed. The overall goals for outcomes and decision support data are to improve quality, reduce costs and resource consumption, increase profitability of the organization, and develop an information-based strategic plan. Comparisons of LOS, costs, complications, and mortality cannot be made legitimately without adjusting severity at the patient level. Severity adjustment and clinical case mix permit effective analysis and eliminate practitioners' concerns that "their patients are sicker."

Decision support data facilitate cross-functional analyses to improve patient care processes and outcomes. Decision support data integrate financial and clinical data and provide the opportunity to perform highly sophisticated data analysis, involving predictive outcome management. These data assist healthcare quality managers and executive staff to evaluate current operations and the feasibility of the development of new product lines and services.

Healthcare quality managers coordinate the outcome and decision support data by posing pertinent questions:

- What kinds of comparative analyses will be most important?
- With whom should we compare ourselves?
- How can we be sure the data are really comparable?
- What do we do when the data reveal significant differences in our outcomes and the outcomes of the peer or benchmark?

D. Benchmarking

Where comparison reveals differences, the healthcare organization's management staff can begin to ask questions internally to determine the cause of these variances. The challenge for quality management staff is to display the outcomes data in a meaningful way that will be used by the involved departments or teams. Graphic display of the data enhances understanding and the use of the results.

Benchmarking is the comparison of an organization's or an individual practitioner's results against a reference point. Ideally, the reference point should be a demonstrated best practice. Healthcare quality professionals assist the organization and its practitioners in interpreting benchmarking results. It is important to clarify two very important aspects of benchmarking. The organization or practitioner's actual performance or outcomes always stay the same. However, depending upon to whom the organization or physician is compared, the expected value can change. For instance, an organization's complication rate may only be 6% higher than expected when compared to a selected market. However, the same organization may have an 11% higher-than-expected complication rate when compared to the U.S. average. In other words, the comparison value and the magnitude of difference change.

Healthcare quality professionals need to ask the right questions to find out how their organization works, and then ask more questions to compare it to the best performers. The goal is to identify how to improve the organization's outcomes, not to identify the differences between it and the benchmarking partner. It is important to be able to take the benchmarking data and provide the pertinent results to the right audience. When variance is identified, the department or service involved must ask the following questions:

- What are we doing?
- How are we doing it?
- What is the measure of how well we do it?
- Why are we looking for improvement?

Directed and focused questions help managers to identify performance gaps.

Benchmarking needs to be an essential element of clinical pathway development to ensure the highest-cost, highest-opportunity DRGs are prioritized. Data-driven internal and external comparisons not only help to set best practices, but also appeal to healthcare professionals by providing objective data for clinical pathway development. In general, three steps must be followed when benchmarking clinical pathways:

1. Identify high-resource-utilization DRGs.
2. Assess internal variability.
3. Benchmark against external sources.

Table 1-3 illustrates examples of benchmarking projects.

Table 1-3. Examples of Benchmarking Projects

Type of Benchmarking	Example Topic	Measures
Internal	Cesarean section rate	Physician A vs. B vs. C, etc.; physician group practice A vs. B, etc.; physicians vs. midwives
Internal	Time to antibiotic for XYZ infection	Emergency dept. vs. unit A vs. unit B, etc.; emergency dept. vs. urgent care setting
External	Use of ACE inhibitors with acute myocardial infarction	Health system or proprietary database performance of all hospitals vs. region vs. similar size hospital vs. your hospital
External	Central line-associated blood stream infection rates	Your unit's vs. National Nosocomial Infection Surveillance (NNIS) data for similar units. Can compare by quartile or median rates (industry standard).
Zero-incidence	Wrong site/wrong procedure/wrong person surgery	Your hospital's incidence vs. zero incidence

Benchmarking enables an organization to set a target or goal for its performance improvement activities. It is up to the performance improvement team to determine whether it wants to be "average" (the industry standard) or to raise the bar to a much higher level of performance. Obviously, the goal is to improve performance, so the goal depends on the level of current performance and the commitment of the performance team and healthcare providers. One of the most critical decisions an organization makes when launching a benchmarking initiative is selecting the source of its benchmarking comparative data. Healthcare quality professionals often coordinate an organization's benchmarking efforts. Most healthcare regulatory agencies require benchmarking as part of a comprehensive quality improvement program.

Potential data sources for benchmarking include the following:

- Government data available from CMS and state government agencies

- Alliances such as large healthcare systems (partnership organizations often provide data extrapolation for their members, frequently providing databases for internal and external benchmarking)
- Those state peer review organizations and state hospital associations that offer free benchmarking opportunities for hospitals within their state
- For-profit database companies that offer software that helps hospitals or organizations extrapolate and compile their own benchmark data, or that provide benchmarking data through a centralized database compiled by the company. These data also are reported to regulatory agencies upon request such as the Joint Commission's ORYX and Core Measures, CMS' OASIS, and the National Association for Quality Assurance's HEDIS requirement.

VII. Systematic Healthcare Quality

A. Development of a Quality Information System

Healthcare professionals are constantly challenged to sift and interpret the vast amount of data available and then distinguish what is relevant from what is irrelevant to plan a course of action. For example, a nurse in an intensive care unit may be monitoring the patient's electrocardiogram readings and vital signs, and based upon his or her interpretation of the relative importance of those ongoing data, the nurse must choose a course of action that will ultimately have an effect on the patient's opportunity for improved functional status. So, too, quality-of-care data must be interpreted in order to make informed decisions related to quality-of-care outcomes. The keys to all quality improvement activities are the collection of meaningful data and the communication of useful information. The trick is to communicate the right information the right way at the right time to the right people.

There is a distinction between data and information:

- *Data* are the abstract representation of things, facts, concepts, and instructions that are stored in a defined format and structure on a passive medium (e.g., paper, computer, microfilm).
- *Information*, on the other hand, is obtained when data are translated into results and statements that are useful for decision making. For information to be meaningful, data must be considered within the context of how they were obtained and how they are to be used (Quality Measurement and Management Project, 1991).

An information distribution system must be developed whereby effective processes are identified for information gathering and dissemination (Tweed-Weber, Inc., 1992). An organization must

- identify who needs to know the information (this may include various stakeholders like senior management, board members, customers, physicians, etc.)
- determine what information they need to know in order to make decisions related to improving the quality of care
- develop a system whereby the right people receive the right information at the right time in the right way.

The Quality Measurement and Management Project (1991, p. 28) has developed seven basic concepts related to quality management information:

- Healthcare data must be carefully defined and systematically collected and analyzed in their full context before they can be useful in quality management.
- There are tremendous amounts of healthcare data and information available, but not all of it is useful for quality management.
- Mature quality management information revolves around clearly established patterns of care, not individual cases. Patterns identify a consistent process, which can be studied and improved.
- Most quality indicators currently available are useful only as indicators of potential problems and not as definitive measures of quality.
- Multiple measures of quality need to be integrated to provide a clear picture of quality of care in an institution or managed care organization.
- Developing outcomes information without monitoring the process of care, when warranted, is inefficient because it cannot lead directly to quality improvements.
- Cost and quality are inseparable issues.

B. Strategy for Interpretation and Utilization of Information

Based upon the seven concepts, the Quality Measurement and Management Project devised a seven-step strategy for the interpretation and utilization of quality-of-care information (Bader & Bohr, 1991).

Step 1. Planning and Organizing for Data Collection, Interpretation, and Use

Advance planning for collection and utilization of internally and externally generated data leads to a greater likelihood of success. Anticipating barriers, identifying responsibilities, and laying the groundwork for multidisciplinary collaboration can more smoothly guide the process toward improvement. In addition, a data dictionary defining all the data elements and calculations of indicators can be an invaluable element in improving the communication of information.

Step 2. Verifying and Correcting Data

The purpose of verifying data is to identify limitations of the data, to provide an opportunity for correcting the data, to identify opportunities for improving internal systems that lead to better data, and to review the data in order to become familiar with it.

Step 3. Identifying and Presenting Potentially Important Findings

The first step in this process is to perform preliminary data analysis, often descriptive analyses. When conducting this type of analysis, Bader and Bohr (1991) recommend that several questions be addressed:

- How do these data compare with other organizations' (as with mortality rates) or with previously trended internal data (for example, nosocomial rates)?
- What is the trend over time? Is it static, improving, or worsening?
- How are data likely to be interpreted (or misinterpreted)?
- Is there an opportunity for improvement?
- Who should receive the data? For what purpose?

Data must be translated into meaningful information. Several techniques are utilized to present information in a clear and concise manner. Bader and Bohr (1991) describe the use of tables, graphics, and visuals.

Tables are the most common format for presenting information. By highlighting the most pertinent information, the reader can quickly and efficiently hone in on key information. For tables to be most effective, they should be understandable and utilize minimal abbreviations or jargon. They should have columns clearly identified, with specific findings highlighted with boldface type, underlining, or other distinguishing marks.

Graphics and visuals provide a "snapshot" of where the organization is; where the variations lie; the relative importance of identified problems; and the impact, if any, of changes that have been instituted (Brassard, 1988).

Common graphical techniques include

- Pareto diagram/chart: prioritizes a series of problems or possible causes of problems
- histogram: illustrates the variability or distribution of data
- scatter diagram: displays possible cause and effect; they illustrate whether one variable might have an impact upon another variable and can illustrate the strength of that impact
- run chart: used to monitor processes over time
- control chart: used to statistically illustrate upper and lower limits of a process and the variation of an organization's process within those limits
- stratification: breaks down single values into meaningful categories or classification to focus on improvement opportunities or corrective action (Brassard, 1988).

In recent years, organizations have developed "dashboards" to represent key management and performance indicators. They can be used as data-mining tools to synchronize and synthesize vast amounts of data into visual representations. Dashboards can be used for analyzing and forecasting various organizational systems.

Step 4. Continuing to Study and Develop Recommendations for Change

If further study of the data is warranted, a variety of methods are available. These include variation analysis, review of additional data, retrospective medical reviews, and process analysis (Bader & Bohr, 1991). Variation analysis seeks an explanation for statistically significant differences in the data. These differences may be due to clinical factors, patient characteristics, data collection (such as sampling characteristics), or organizational characteristics (such as staffing).

Additional data may need to be collected and reviewed to completely understand the variations in data. For instance, a hospital may show a steady increase in mortality rates. Additional data related to hospital case mix, diagnostic categories, mortality within a specified time from date of hospital admission, and other hospital characteristics may be utilized to fully interpret the data.

Focused/intensive retrospective review refers to those activities whereby processes or outcomes are utilizing preestablished criteria or indicators. Findings may be presented in peer review or other settings.

Process analysis refers to a method of analyzing data using industrial quality improvement techniques. Process analysis occurs whenever a group of individuals diagrams a healthcare process. The group then measures process variations and looks for ways to improve the process and, therefore, improve the administrative or clinical outcome.

Step 5. Taking Action

"Taking action" implies that the individuals, teams, departments, and committees are empowered to make decisions and implement changes based on the information discovered by analyzing the data. Actions may occur in several forms: education and training of staff, education and/or reporting of findings to outside vendors or the public, changes in organizational or departmental policies and processes, and changes in practice patterns.

Step 6. Monitoring Performance

Monitoring performance is actually monitoring the impact and effectiveness of the quality improvement action and involves the collection of additional data.

Questions to be considered include these (Bader & Bohr, 1991):

- Have the proposed changes actually been implemented? To what extent?
- How could compliance with the changes be enhanced?
- What effect are the changes having on patient outcomes? Are these desirable effects?
- Should the changes be modified and then tested further, communicated on a wider scale, tested for a longer period of time before drawing conclusions, or ended because they are ineffective?

Step 7. Communicating Results

Communication is an integral component of each of the previous steps. Striving for healthcare quality is a journey. Quality improvement begins with the communication of where an organization is and where it is going.

Bader and Bohr (1991) delineate three basic barriers to the interpretation and utilization of information: human factors, statistical factors, and organizational factors.

- Human factors include fear of the data, resentment of external data; unrealistic expectations about data (including the myth that all data must be perfect); and lack of training related to planning, organizing, and analyzing data.
- Statistical factors include flawed data, untimely data, poorly displayed data, and data that are difficult to integrate with other organizational data.
- Organizational factors include data overload; poor data retrieval system; lack of resources (time, people, money); and poor relationships among administration, physicians, and staff.

VIII. Management Information Systems

A management information system (MIS) can contain both the manual and the automated methods that provide information for decision making. Other names for an MIS, which are used interchangeably, include data-processing structure, medical information system, hospital information system, or decision support system. The term, as it is commonly used, refers to an automated or computerized system. Information plays a key role in decision making in each stage of the management process. Whether a staff member or manager is trying to establish goals, estimate resources, allocate resources, evaluate a quality improvement process, or monitor a system, access to accurate and timely information is an ongoing requirement of any MIS. The quality of judgments and decisions is directly correlated with availability and reliability of data and its synthesis into information.

The choices for the design or flow of information are so important that they actually can be a determining factor in the survival of a patient or an organization.

Although accurate and timely healthcare information is what should provide the rationale for management decisions, this often is not the case. Information, according to O'Rourke and Bader (1993), often is incomplete, confusing, and not sufficiently relevant to the organization's mission, strategic goals, or customer and stakeholder needs when it is presented in many governing body reports. These authors make a strong point that organizations should clarify the difference between data and information; and that data must be carefully selected, validated, and formatted to make them useful. This often is easier to mandate than to accomplish. However, the goal remains that governing body reports contain only the critical information needed for effective decision making. The achievement of this goal would eliminate healthcare data being presented as a pile of computer printouts and various fragmented reports.

According to O'Rourke and Bader (1993), the information contained in data helps leaders to

- assess how well the mission and values are being achieved, by applying quantitative measures to the ideals espoused in their mission and vision statements
- understand changes in community needs, financial resources, and technology
- develop a vision and evaluate program achievements
- identify the need for policy implementation effectiveness
- prioritize strategic goals, including programs, to support or discontinue
- judge progress toward strategic goals and objectives
- weigh long-term and short-term financial viability
- weigh the impact of budgetary decisions on quality of care/services
- determine priorities for continuous improvements
- monitor aspects of organizational performance and take corrective action
- understand the mechanism for physician appointment and recredentialing, while knowing their performance review process is effective
- decide on individual credentialing recommendations effectively
- determine goals for improving the health status of the community
- evaluate the effectiveness of programs designed to improve health
- defend the organization's resources, efficiency, and effectiveness based on accurate information
- help the governing body to evaluate and improve its performance.

A. Purposes of Information Systems

Information systems can be used to support a variety of activities within healthcare organizations. Those areas commonly supported include quality improvement, cost control and productivity, patient registration, utilization management, program planning and evaluation, external reporting, research, and education. An MIS can identify problems, provide evidence to lead to solutions, and evaluate the results of implemented strategies (Burton & Hoy, 1993).

Information systems can be grouped into the following: clinical information systems, administrative support information systems, and decision support systems.

1. Clinical Information Systems

Designed to support direct patient care processes, automated clinical information systems have great potential for analyzing and improving the quality of patient care.

Barriers to healthcare leaders' and healthcare organizations' implementation of MIS include normal resistance to change, the mindset that patients can best be tended to by the human mind, lack of exposure to information science and computers in healthcare educational and training programs, and inadequate resources. A recent study found that, on average, Florida hospitals use only 38% of the available clinical healthcare information technologies associated with the six IOM care aims (Burke, Menachemi, & Brooks, 2005).

Currently, expanded clinical information systems in use include medical records and their retrieval systems; computer-assisted medical decision making for history and physicals and antibiotic selection; and clinical application programs for health risk programs and health maintenance organization encounter data.

From a managed care perspective, Rontal (1993) outlines the following criteria as needed for an MIS: appropriate use, place of service, specific procedures, preventive care, cost-effectiveness, patient satisfaction, chronic illness management, access to care, and patient education. Also needed are outcomes of care for mortality, morbidity, complications, readmissions, quality of life, and disability. Clinical information systems often depend on integration with administrative information systems for some data.

2. Administrative Support Information Systems

Administrative support information systems aid day-to-day operations in healthcare organizations, including

1. *Financial information systems*
    - payroll
    - accounts payable
    - patient accounting
    - cost accounting
    - budgeting.
2. *Human resources information systems*
    - employee record
    - position management
    - labor analysis
    - turnover and absenteeism.
3. *Office automation systems*
    - word processing
    - electronic mail
    - scheduling
    - facsimile transmitting
    - electronic spreadsheets.

3. Decision Support Systems

Decision support systems deal with strategic planning functions (see Section VI, Decision Support, Risk Adjustment, Data Interpretation, and Benchmarking; also see Module Two: Strategy and Leadership, for more details). Included in this area are

- strategic planning and marketing
- resource allocation
- performance evaluation and monitoring
- product evaluation and services
- medical management (e.g., evidence-based practice, clinical pathways).

B. Implementation of a Quality Management Information System

1. Evaluating Systems

The following is a checklist of issues to consider when evaluating various computerization options:

- Does the system provide for capture, storage, and retrieval of clinical and financial information from a variety of sources (e.g., medical records, admission/discharge/transfer, billing, laboratory, pharmacy, blood bank, operating room schedule, and radiology)?
- Does the system interface with the organization's existing information systems?
- Does the system allow for the establishment of "triggers" or thresholds for important measures of performance and signal an alert when these thresholds have been exceeded?
- Does the system have critical alerts such as abnormal laboratory values, drug interactions, and others to promote patient safety?
- Does the system have "rules-based" processing (i.e., the system automatically provides a complete list of cases that meet or fail criteria)?
- Is the system flexible enough to allow for both concurrent and retrospective reviews?
- Does the system support Joint Commission and other accreditation and regulatory reporting requirements?
- Does the system have the capability for data mining reporting, and/or statistical analysis?
- Does the system allow for multiple users to access the same programs at the same time?
- It is an "open operating system" (i.e., one that enables users to operate on a variety of different hardware platforms)?
- Does the system have networking capabilities?
- Will the system display data in graphic form?
- Is there the capability for drill-down analysis of underlying causes of outcomes?
- Does the system allow access to reports via a secure Intranet Web site within the organization?

2. Buy or Build?

The following is a checklist of issues to consider when making the choice between developing an in-house quality management system versus purchasing a system developed by an outside vendor:

- Does the organization have the in-house expertise to build the system, database software, analytic tools, and hardware for such a project? If not, how much money and time will have to be invested to procure this expertise?
- Do either data processing or quality management staff have the full industry knowledge required to build an automated information system (architecture, nomenclature, and other national standards)?
- Can staff provide documentation, training, support, and maintenance for the system on an ongoing basis? If so, will changing priorities interfere with the sustainability of the program?
- What happens if the staff member who designed the program leaves the facility? Will the organization still be able to support the system?

- Is there enough expertise to build the system with the broad picture in mind? Is there a true understanding of the future data demands of accreditors and regulators, third-party payers, employers, and other outsiders' information demands?
- Are resources available to keep the program up to date in an ever-changing environment?
- Can the time of a programmer or coordinator be dedicated for an extended period of time to build such an application for quality improvement (including various functions such as credentialing, profiling, etc.)?
- What would be gained by being part of an established vendor network or user group addressing the needs of credentialing and quality improvement?
- Is it more cost-effective to develop such applications in-house or would the facility be better served by purchasing software dedicated to these needs?

C. Federal HIT Initiatives

The need to accelerate the adoption of HIT has been widely recognized and was singled out as a key goal by the Health Care Delivery and Information Technology (HCDIT) Subcommittee of the President's Information Technology Advisory Committee (2004). Recent studies have suggested that the quality of healthcare can improve with the appropriate use of technology (Bates & Gawande, 2003; Weiner, et al., 2003). These studies specifically highlight the need to facilitate the transmission of clinical information that is contained in the medical record between healthcare providers. A second goal identified by the HCDIT subcommittee is the use of HIT to achieve substantial economic and social benefits (i.e., to reduce medical errors, eliminate unproductive healthcare expenditures, and to improve quality of care).

A lack of standards has hindered the adoption of information technology tools in the healthcare industry (Bates & Gawande, 2003). However, an effort by the National Committee on Vital and Health Statistics (NCVHS) to standardize formats and data for the electronic exchange of patient health record information is encouraging (NCVHS, 2002). In addition, other organizations and task forces are working on international protocols and frameworks for data exchanges between heterogeneous systems in the healthcare industry. The industry Health Level 7 (HL7; www.hl7.org) and XML Special Interest Groups have been leaders in defining electronic health record (EHR) standards. As these standards evolve, it is more likely that comprehensive EHRs will be developed and shared among all the providers in the healthcare system. It should be noted that EHRs sometimes are referred to as personal health records (PHR). There is a distinction between the two types of records, in that PHRs are geared more toward consumers and EHRs pertain to those records used by healthcare providers.

Federal support is increasing with the announcement in 2004 of the U.S. Department of Health and Human Services 10-year plan to create a new national health information infrastructure. This will include an EHR for every American and a new network to link health records nationwide. David J. Brailer, MD PhD, National Coordinator for the HIT initiatives, was appointed to lead the effort. Clearly, software vendors and information technology departments within healthcare organizations will need to plan for the impact of these new initiatives. It is very likely that there will be a need for system changes and demands that data interchange among organizations follow the emerging standards.

Advances in HIT will facilitate an evolving quality agenda in coming years. HIT provides the infrastructure to enhance patient safety, transparency, public reporting, and pay for performance.

IX. Quality Improvement Study Design and Analysis

A. Getting Started on Quality Improvement Projects

Healthcare quality professionals and their quality improvement teams prioritize performance improvement activities based on the quantitative and qualitative data available to them. The initiatives that have the most opportunity for improvement should be tackled first. Usually, the initiatives selected will focus on core processes, high-risk processes, high-risk patients and populations, high-risk medications, or high-risk actions/interventions. The level of risk is based on the potential consequences of injury or harm to patients. Managing high-risk patients and processes will significantly affect morbidity and mortality.

Examples of high-risk processes include

- core processes: admission, transfer, discharge
- high-risk processes: medication delivery/administration, surgery
- high-risk patients: patients with reduced renal function, patients who are immunocompromised, neonates, patients in critical care units
- high-risk medications: heparin, insulin, chemotherapy, opiates
- high-risk actions/interventions: blood transfusions, use of restraints, extracorporeal circulation (White, 2004).

Key steps to implementing quality improvement activities are as follows (Rosati, 2003; White, 2004). These steps ensure success of the quality improvement models described earlier in this module.

1. Ensure leadership support and commitment for the quality improvement initiative.
2. Assess priority and feasibility of initiative based on risk, resources, leadership support, and organizational strategies.
3. Identify the aim of the initiative and include the topic, process, or problem to be improved (have a good rationale).
4. Convene an interdisciplinary team of content and process experts with all key disciplines as participants (involve all of the right people and have a champion for the change).
5. Utilize tools and techniques to analyze processes, best practices, research, and consensus-based evidence for the desired change.
6. Develop the change to be implemented and add timelines and accountability for the project.
7. Identify the measure(s) to demonstrate that the change has resulted in improvement; set performance goals.
8. Educate staff on the desired change.
9. Implement and test the change via the redesigned processes.
10. Collect, analyze, and evaluate data on the redesigned process.
11. Make additional changes based on findings, and disseminate to all areas.
12. Report and display results to reward staff on improvements.
13. Continue to monitor performance to ensure that the change is sustained.
14. Compare performance internally and externally.
15. Celebrate successes internally and externally.

B. Data and Data Management

There are two general types of data: measurement/continuous and count/categorical. Ordinal data are a form of categorical data. Methods of sampling, data collection, and analysis are different for each type or level of data. This distinction is critical because quality improvement work involves both types of data and their associated statistics. This is one of the greatest sources of confusion for people new to quality improvement and data analysis.

The data levels are *categorical* (nominal and ordinal) and *continuous* (interval and ratio).

1. Categorical

Nominal. Nominal data also are called *count, discrete,* or *qualitative* data. In statistical process control (SPC), these are known as *attributes data*. Binary data are categorical data with only two possibilities (e.g., gender). Numerical values can be assigned to each category as a label to facilitate data analysis, but this is purely arbitrary and has no quantitative value. There is no order to these data. Examples of nominal scale data are as follows:

Nominal Variables	Values
Surgical patients	Preoperative Postoperative
Gender	Male Female
Patient education	Attended video session Did not attend video session

Ordinal. For this type of data, characteristics are put into categories and are rank-ordered. Assignment to the categories is not arbitrary. Examples of ordinal scale data are as follows:

Ordinal Variables	Values
Nursing staff rank	1. Nurse Level I 2. Nurse Level II 3. Nurse Level III
Education	1. Diploma/Associate Degree 2. BS 3. MS 4. PhD
Attitude toward research scale (a Likert scale)	1. Strongly agree 2. Agree 3. Neutral 4. Disagree 5. Strongly disagree

2. Continuous

Continuous or "measured" data are measured on scales that theoretically have no gaps. The SPC term for this is *variables data*. There are two subtypes of continuous data: interval and ratio.

- *Interval*. For interval-level data, the distance between each point is equal (e.g., the values on a Fahrenheit thermometer).
- *Ratio*. For ratio-level data, the distance between each point is equal and there is a true zero.

Measurement/continuous data often can be converted to count/categorical data. For example, the number of pounds lost by a hemodialysis patient during treatment in relationship to his or her desired or "dry weight" is measurement data. If Mr. Jones was admitted at 170 lb and was discharged at his dry weight of 165 lb, then he measured a 5-lb weight loss. If the nurse manager wanted to know the number of patients finishing their treatments at their "dry weight" for the entire day, then this information would be an example of count data and would be converted into "yes/no" format.

A critical issue is whether the right data are measured or counted. A common criticism of quality improvement activities is that readily available data, such as patient visits, deaths, infections, falls, cost, and laboratory tests, are analyzed for improvement specifically because the data are easy to retrieve.

3. Statistical Power of Different Data Types

Categorical data are the least powerful statistically, whereas continuous data have the most power. The practical meaning of this when comparing patient outcomes after process change is that fewer data points (and fewer subjects) are needed if data in continuous form are collected, assuming that the researcher has a choice. For example, when dealing with blood pressure, a healthcare quality manager might collect the data by categorizing subjects as either hypertensive or nonhypertensive, or by recording the measured levels of systolic and diastolic pressure. The latter form is more powerful and allows more flexibility in data analysis.

When a quality improvement project is designed, each step must be planned and accountability assigned. Each organization should adopt a quality improvement model that facilitates performance improvement and is in alignment with its mission, vision, core values, goals, and strategic plan.

C. Data Collection Plan

The development of a comprehensive data collection plan should include these steps:

- Determine the who, what, when, where, how, and why.
- Structure the design.
- Choose and develop the sampling method.
- Determine and conduct the necessary training.
- Delegate responsibilities.
- Facilitate interdepartmental/cross-functional coordination.
- Forecast the budget requirements.
- Conduct pilot procedures for the forms and the data collection process.

Data collection can be both expensive and time-consuming for any organization. Just enough data should be collected; avoid overmeasurement in terms of both number of measures and frequency of measurement and analysis. Try to prevent duplicate data collection efforts among different groups and departments. Always pilot a new data collection process, even if it is new only to the organization.

D. Basic Sampling Designs

A *population* (*N*) is the total aggregate or group (e.g., all cases that meet a designated set of criteria for practitioners, all patients who have died at a particular hospital, or all registered nurses with a tenure of 10 years or more).

Sampling makes research more feasible because it allows researchers to sample a portion of the population to represent the entire population (*n*). A sample usually is selected from the accessible population; that is, the population that is available.

Sampling has several purposes, the main ones being to

- provide a logical way of making statements about a larger group based on a smaller group
- allow researchers to make inferences or generalize from the sample to the population if the selection process has been random and systematic (i.e., unbiased).

1. Types of Sampling

a. Probability

Probability sampling requires every element in the population to have an equal or random chance of being selected for inclusion in the sample. The following are subsets of probability sampling.

Simple random sampling. Each individual in the sampling frame (all subjects in the population) has an equal chance of being chosen. For example, pulling a name out of a hat containing all possible names.

Systematic sampling. After randomly selecting the first case, this method involves drawing every *n*th element from a population. For example, picking every third name from a list of possible names.

Stratified random sampling. A subpopulation is a *stratum*, and *strata* are two or more homogeneous subpopulations. After the population has been divided into strata, each member of a stratum has an equal probability of being selected. Examples of strata include sex, ethnicity, patients with particular diseases, or patients living in certain parts of the country.

Cluster sampling. This method requires that the population be divided into groups, or clusters. For example, if a researcher is studying medical students, she or he may not have individuals' names but may have a list of medical schools in the area. The sample may therefore be randomly derived from this list of medical schools.

b. Nonprobability

Nonprobability sampling provides no way of estimating the probability that each element will be included in the sample. When this approach is used, the results will be representative of the sample only and cannot be generalized to the available population. The following are subsets of nonprobability sampling.

Convenience sampling. This approach allows the use of any available group of subjects. Because of the lack of randomization in this sampling method, the subjects may be atypical in some way. Sending a survey to a list of members of an elder organization may not reflect the opinions of all elders, for instance. Convenience sampling may include all patients at an organization who are undergoing a certain procedure over a 12-month period.

Snowball sampling. This is a subtype of convenience sampling. This method involves subjects suggesting other subjects for inclusion in the study, so that the sampling process gains momentum. This type of sampling process gains subjects who are difficult to identify, but are known to others because of an informal network.

Selection bias may be present in all convenience sampling because the selected subjects may not accurately reflect the population of interest.

Purposive or judgment sampling. This method selects a particular group or groups based on certain criteria. This method is subjective, and the researcher uses his or her judgment to decide who is representative of the population. Using a group of nurses because the researcher believes that they represent a cross section of women is an example of this type of sampling.

Expert sampling. This is a type of purposive sampling that involves selecting experts in a given area because of their access to the information relevant to the study. Expert sampling is used in the Delphi technique, in which several rounds of questionnaires are distributed on the selected topic and sent to experts to elicit their responses, and are sent out again after the initial data analysis. The goal is to achieve fairly rapid group consensus. A conference planning team is an example if they utilize the Delphi method to identify potential program content that would be of interest to those in the same professions for an upcoming conference.

Quota sampling. In this type of sampling, the researcher makes a judgment decision about the best type of sample for the investigation. That is, the researcher prespecifies characteristics of the sample to increase its representativeness. The researcher identifies strata of the population and determines the proportions of elements needed from the various segments of the population. Stratification may be based on any demographic, such as age or ethnicity.

2. Sample Size

Many factors may influence the determination of sample size, such as the research purpose, the design, the level of confidence desired, the anticipated degree of difference between study groups, and the size of the population. Depending on these factors, a small or large sample size may be appropriate. However, with the exception of case studies, the larger the sample, the more valid and accurate the study, because a larger sample size is more likely to be more representative of the population. Thus, the larger the sample, the smaller the sample error of the mean, which is a measure of fluctuation of a statistic from one sample to another drawn from the same population. Also, as the actual difference between study groups gets smaller, the size of the sample required to detect the difference gets larger. Outcomes that are measured on a continuous scale and/or using repeated measures require fewer subjects than do categorical outcomes. Using too large a sample to answer a research question is a waste of time and resources.

E. Data Analysis

1. Reporting

The reporting, analysis, and ultimate interpretation of data are what make them meaningful. Good presentation of data creates interest and enhances understanding. Data should be reported and analyzed on a regular basis. In this process, it is important to validate that the data were collected accurately. Data should be displayed in a format that is easily understood, and a brief summary should be provided. Those involved in the process being monitored should be asked to help with the analysis. There should be an analysis of variances and identification of unexpected patterns among caregivers, services, patients, etc. If there are trends, people should be asked to identify possible causes and solutions.

2. Importance of Context

To effectively interpret data, it is essential to provide a contextual background. Because most people are visually oriented, a graph should be used to display the data. A table of values should accompany the graph. There should be an explanation as to specifics regarding the data collection (i.e., how, when, and where the data were collected; and from whom they were obtained). There also should be a report summarizing the meaning of the values and how they were computed. If outliers were removed from the sample, that should be stated. The time-order of the data collection should be included in the presentation to determine whether a pattern exists.

3. Variation

Use of an SPC chart is helpful in understanding and interpreting a function or process. The performance of functions or processes varies over time. This variation is expected and predictable and is referred to as *random* or *common cause* variation. A process is said to be "in control" if the variation is within the computed upper and lower limits and no trends are evident. There is no need to take action if a process is in control. *Special cause* variation occurs when activity falls outside the control limits or there is an obvious nonrandom pattern around the central line. This type of variation should be interpreted as a trend and investigated.

4. Trend Identification

When a trend is identified, an investigation should be initiated to determine the cause. In some cases, an interdisciplinary team may be convened to further analyze and improve the process. The team should use CQI principles and tools (e.g., histograms, flowcharts, Pareto charts, cause-and-effect diagrams, run charts). After a thorough analysis of the process has been completed, the team should select and implement appropriate corrective measures.

F. Statistical Analysis and Interpretation of Findings

1. Measurement Tools

Instruments are the devices that healthcare quality professionals and researchers use to obtain and record the data received from the subjects. These instruments can include questionnaires, rating scales, interview transcripts, and the like. It is critical to use the most credible tools possible, that is, those with proven reliability and validity.

2. Reliability

Reliability is the extent to which an experiment, test, or measuring procedure yields the same results on repeated trials. For example, a scale that measures a person's weight as 110 lb one minute and then yields a reading of 160 lb a minute later would be considered unreliable and not capable of meeting the standards for accuracy or consistency.

a. Reliability Coefficient

The stability of an instrument is derived through procedures referred to as *test-retest reliability*. This is done by administering the test to a sample of individuals on two occasions, and then comparing the scores obtained. The comparison results in a reliability coefficient, the numerical index of how reliable the test is. The closer the coefficient is to 1.0, the more reliable the tool. In general, reliability coefficients of ≥0.70 are considered acceptable, although ≥0.80 is desired. The reliability coefficient can be determined by evaluating the internal consistency of a measure. This refers to the degree to which the subparts of an instrument are all measuring the same attribute or dimension. The "split-half" technique is one of the oldest methods for assessing internal consistency of an instrument and can be done by hand. It correlates scores on half of the measure with scores on the other half.

The concept of *reliability by equivalence* is established by comparing scores from the various versions of the instrument that have been developed (e.g., parallel forms or alternate forms of a test). This is used to compare different translations of a measurement tool or different forms of the CPHQ examination, for instance.

b. Interrater Reliability

This concept refers to the degree to which two raters, operating independently, assign the same ratings in the context of observational research or in coding qualitative materials. The monitoring of the accuracy of a patient classification system entails interrater reliability. The staff that monitors the system must be able to assign the same classification to the same patient to ensure reliability of their monitoring. Interrater reliability is frequently reported as a degree of concordance, or Cohen's kappa.

3. Validity

Validity is the degree to which an instrument measures what it is intended to measure. Validity usually is more difficult to establish than reliability. The validity and reliability of an instrument are not wholly independent of each other. An instrument that is not reliable cannot possibly be valid. However, an instrument that is reliable does not have to have validity. For example, a thermometer is a reliable instrument, but it is not valid for measuring height.

a. Content (Face) Validity

This is the degree to which the instrument adequately represents the universe of content. Content validity, although necessary, is not a sufficient indication that the instrument measures what it is intended to measure. For example, a panel of rehabilitation specialists evaluated the functional independence measure (FIM) tool and identified that it measured the key aspects of functional independence. On the other hand, a survey designed to measure patient satisfaction with the primary care provider would be considered inadequate in terms of content validity if it failed to cover the major dimensions of access, waiting time, and practitioner-patient interaction.

Content validity includes judgments by experts or respondents about the degree to which the test appears to measure the relevant construct.

b. Construct Validity

This concept refers to the degree to which an instrument measures the theoretical construct or trait that it was designed to measure. For example, severity adjustment scales are tools for measuring staffing needs. Risk adjustment scales are tools for predicting the probability of outcomes such as morbidity and mortality. If a previously used satisfaction tool had demonstrated validity, a new, abbreviated tool can be compared to the "old" tool to determine whether the new tool has construct validity. Similarly, two functional status health outcome measures could be compared, such as the SF-36 and SF-12 instruments.

c. Criterion-Related Validity

This concept refers to the extent that the score on the instrument can be related to a criterion (the behavior that the instrument is supposed to predict). Criterion-related validity can be either predictive or concurrent, depending on when the criterion variable is measured. If the criterion variable is obtained at the same time as the measurement under study, *concurrent validity* is assessed. If the criterion measure is obtained at some future time (after the predictor instrument was used), *predictive validity* is assessed. A patient classification system has criterion-related validity, because it predicts staffing needs.

4. Statistical Techniques

The discussion of statistical techniques that follows is in no way a complete account of each topic. Other sources for more information on the various statistical techniques, including Hansen's CAN'T MISS series, are included in the list of Suggested Reading at the end of this section.

a. Measures of Central Tendency

Measures of central tendency are statistical indexes that describe where a set of scores or values of a distribution cluster. *Central* refers to the middle value, and *tendency* refers to the general trend of the numbers. A healthcare quality manager or researcher might ask questions relating to central tendency when answering queries such as, "What is the average LOS for patients with chronic obstructive pulmonary disease?" or "What is the Apgar score of most infants born in the new birthing suites?" The three most common measures of central tendency are the mean, the median, and the mode. The type and distribution of the data determine which measures of central tendency (and spread) are most appropriate.

(1) Mean

The *mean* (*M*) of a set of measurements is the sum of all scores or values divided by the total number of scores. The mean, also known as the average, is the most widely used measure of central tendency in statistical tests of significance.

Example: If five infants had Apgar scores of 7, 8, 8, 9, and 8, the sum of the values should be calculated, and then divided by the total number of infants: $7 + 8 + 8 + 9 + 8 = 40$; $40 \div 5 = 8$; therefore, 8 is the mean.

The mean is the most commonly used of all the measures of central tendency, but it is the most sensitive to extreme scores. In the example given above, if one infant was severely depressed at the time of Apgar scoring and was given a value of 1 instead of 9, the mean then would be 6.4, rather than 8.

It is appropriate to compute the mean for interval or ratio data where variables can be added and the values show a bell-shaped or normal distribution. It also can be used with ordinal variables that have an approximately normal distribution.

(2) Median

The *median* is the measure of central tendency that corresponds to the middle score; that is, the point on a numerical scale above which and below which 50 percent of the cases fall.

To determine the median of data, first arrange the values in rank order. If the total of values is odd, count up (or down) to the middle value. If there are several identical values clustered at the middle, the median is that value. If the total number of values is even, compute the mean of the two middle values.

Example: Consider the following set of values: 2 2 2 3 4 5 6 6 8 9

The median for this set of numbers is 4.5, which is the value that divides the set exactly in half. Note that an important characteristic of the median is that the calculation does not take into account the quantitative values of the individual scores. An example of this notion can be demonstrated in the sample above. If the last value of 9 were increased to the value 84, the median would remain the same as it does not enter into the computation of the median; only the number of values and the values near the midpoint of the distribution enter into the computation. The median, therefore, is not sensitive to extreme scores or statistical outliers. It is appropriate to compute the median for ordinal data, interval, or ratio data, but not for nominal data.

(3) Mode

The *mode* is the score or value that occurs most frequently in a distribution of scores. Of the three measures of central tendency, the mode is the easiest to determine; simply determine which value occurs most often in the data set.

Example: Look at the following distribution of numbers: 30 31 31 32 33 33 33 33 33 34 35 36

It is easy to determine that the mode is 33; the value of 33 appears five times, a higher frequency than for any other number. An easy way to determine the mode is by using a statistical package to run descriptive data frequencies and/or a stem and leaf plot.

In research studies, the mode is seldom the only measure of central tendency reported. Modes are viewed as a quick and easy method of determining an "average," but they tend to be unstable. This instability means that the modes tend to fluctuate widely from sample to sample, even when drawn from the same population. Thus, the mode is reported infrequently, except for describing "typical" values on nominal data. For example, a research report may describe the sample population demographic data as follows: "The typical respondent was a Hispanic man who was married."

b. Measures of Variability

In the preceding section, the purpose of measuring the central tendencies of data was to describe the ways subjects or cases group together. In contrast, the variability looks at the dispersion, or how the measures are spread out. *Variability* may be further defined as the degree to which values on a set of scores differ. For example, it is expected that there would be greater variability of age within a hospital than within a nursing home or a pediatric intensive care unit. Measures of variability should be interpreted as distances on a scale of values, which are unlike averages that are points representing a central value. The three measures of variability that are presented in this review are the range, the standard deviation, and interpercentile measures.

(1) Range

The *range* is the difference between the highest and lowest values in a distribution of scores. Although it indicates the distance on the score scale between the lowest and highest values, the range is best reported as the values themselves and not as the distance between the values.

Example: Test scores for students range from 98 to 60. The range is 98 minus 60, or 38. When the range is reported in research findings, it normally would be written as a maximum and a minimum, without the subtracted value.

Advantages of the range include that it is a quick estimate of variability and that it provides information about the two endpoints of a distribution. Disadvantages of the range include its instability, as it is based on only two scores; its tendency to increase with sample size; and its sensitivity to extreme values.

(2) Standard Deviation

The *standard deviation* (SD), an average of the deviations from the mean, is the most frequently used statistic for measuring the degree of variability in a set of scores. *Standard* refers to the fact that the deviation indicates a group's average spread of scores or values around their mean; *deviation* indicates how much each score is scattered from the mean. The greater the spread of a distribution, the greater the dispersion or variability from the mean; thus, the standard deviation will be a larger value and is said to be heterogeneous. The more the values cluster around the mean, the smaller the amount of variability or deviation and the more homogeneous the group is said to be; and it will have a smaller standard deviation. The standard bell curve illustrates this measure of variability; see **Figure 1-4**. A histogram can be used to display data distribution and to determine if the data are normally distributed.

Figure 1-4. Normal Distribution

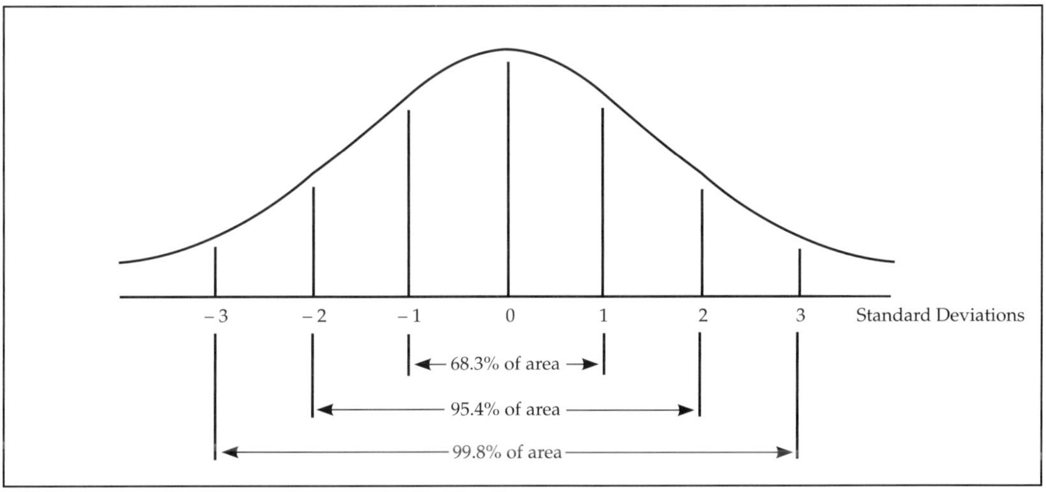

When computing the standard deviation, as with the mean, all of the scores or values in a distribution are taken into consideration. Use of the standard deviation is most appropriate with normally distributed interval or ratio scale data. Standard deviations (and means) also may be calculated for normally distributed values from a broad ordinal scale. Standard deviations can be calculated by hand or with statistical software. The formula is included in the CAN'T MISS series included in the supplemental materials.

Example: The researcher may compare coping-scale scores for two groups of patients, with each group having a different ethnic background. Although each distribution demonstrated a mean score of 30, the standard deviations were computed at 3 and 8, respectively. The investigator could conclude that although the means were alike, one sample was more homogeneous (or had less variance) in its coping skills.

c. Interpercentile Measures

Although there are several interpercentile measures of variability, the most common is the *interquartile range,* a stable measure of variability based on excluding extreme scores and using only middle cases. The interquartile range is more stable than the range and is determined by lining up the measures in order of size and then dividing the array into quarters. The range of scores that includes the middle 50% of the scores is the interquartile range; that is, the range between scores comprising the lowest quartile, or quarter, and the highest quartile. The interquartile range demonstrates how the middle 50% of the distribution is scattered. The first quartile ends at the 25th percentile. Interquartile range values often are presented in "box plots."

Example: Growth charts are one of the most commonly used interpercentile measures. Normal growth is represented by measurements between the 25th and 75th percentiles on the National Center for Health Statistics growth charts.

Example: Clinical pathways should be developed based on the interquartile range of the designated population. Paths should be designed around the average patient, or those in the middle quartiles.

5. Tests of Statistical Significance

Significance tests are categorized as either *parametric* or *nonparametric*. Parametric tests are used with data measured on a continuous scale (i.e., interval or ratio data, which are also known as variables data). Nonparametric tests are used with categorical (attributes) data and should be used with ordinal data, especially if the ordinal categories have a small range of possible values or a nonnormal distribution. **Table 1-4** summarizes statistical options for each type of data.

Table 1-4. Statistical Options for Different Data Types

Type	Categorical	Ordinal	Continuous
a.k.a.	SPC: "attribute"; nominal; discrete; binary (0/1)	Ordinal categorical	SPC: "variables" measured
Examples	Gender; vital status; ethnicity	Age in categories; functional independence measure (FIM) items; patient satisfaction	Age; FIM total; charges; LOS
Usually reported as	Percentage in each category	Percentage in each category (but not always)	Mean; median; min, max; percentiles
Usual statistical test of differences between groups	Chi square (χ^2)	χ^2 for most scales; *t* tests may be appropriate (>6 levels) if there is a broad scale between groups and data are normally distributed.	*t* tests
Control chart*	*p* if rate > 1/100 *u* if 1/1000 < rate < 1/100 *c* if rate < 1/1000	Depends on scale, data distribution and whether regrouped	χ & S; χ bar & R; median and range; individuals
Rules of thumb for sample sizes per plotted point	For *p* charts; +/− 40 common events; up to 200 for rarer events	(see *p* chart rules)	Calculate mean based on 2–10 randomly selected values (3–4 optimal)
Usual regression technique†	Logistic	Logistic (if regrouped as 0/1 outcome)	"Ordinary least squares"

**Most commonly used type; lists not exhaustive*
†Regression is preferred method for simultaneous control of numerous "demographic" variables (e.g., sex, age, ethnicity, severity) and is most commonly used in research settings. To control for the influence of a single demographic variable, consider stratifying the analysis by levels of that demographic variable.

a. Parametric Tests

***t* Test.** A *t* test is used to analyze the difference between two means. When determining whether the difference between two group means is significant, a distinction must be made regarding the two groups. The two groups may be independent, that is, a control group and an experimental group, or they can be dependent, wherein a single group yields pretreatment and post treatment scores.

Example: A healthcare quality manager wants to test the effect of a special educational program on departmental heads' attitudes toward using graphical or visual displays of data in their quality improvement team meeting. Ten of the 20 department heads are randomly assigned to an experiment group, which will be exposed to videos, discussion groups, and lectures on the use of the basic quality control tools and management and planning tools. The remaining 10 department heads compose the control group, which will not receive special instruction on using the tools. At the end of the experiment, both groups are administered a scale measuring attitudes toward using these tools. The two-sample independent *t* test helps the researcher determine if there was a significant statistical difference between the two groups (i.e., whether any difference was due to chance).

Alternatively, if all 20 heads had received the training and had pre- posttraining testing scores, the statistical significance of any changes in average scores would be measured using a "paired sample" *t* test.

Regression analysis. Regression analysis is based on statistical correlations, or associations among variables. A correlation between two variables is used to evaluate the usefulness of a prediction equation. If this correlation were perfect (i.e., $r = 1$ or $r = -1$), it would be possible to make a perfect prediction about the score on one variable, given the score on the other variable. Unfortunately, this is never the case, as there never are perfect correlations; therefore, it never is possible to make perfect predictions. The higher the correlation between variables, the more accurate the degree of prediction. If there was no correlation between two variables (i.e., $r = 0$), knowing the score on one would not help in estimating the score on the other.

In simple linear regression, one variable (x) is used to predict a second variable (y). For example, simple regression can be used to predict weight based on height, or to predict response to a diabetes management program. Regression analysis is performed with the intention of making predictions about phenomena. The ability to make accurate predictions has great implications for quality management in the healthcare industry.

Multiple regression analysis. *Multiple regression analysis* estimates the effects of two or more independent variables (x) on a dependent measure (y). For example, the objective may be to predict intravenous (IV) site infiltration (y) based on predictors (x), which may include osmolarity of the IV solution and addition of an irritating medication, such as potassium, to the IV.

b. Nonparametric Tests

Chi-square (χ^2) tests and categorical (attributes) data. Much of the data collected by healthcare quality managers is counted, not measured. Being counted (e.g., 15 male and 30 female patients in the clinic today) means that many arithmetic operations don't apply (e.g., it is not possible to calculate the average gender of patients). But it certainly is possible to describe the ratio of the counts (e.g., there were twice as many woman as men in the clinic today) or to compare proportions with counted data (50% of male, versus 75% of female patients, came for their appointments today). The chi-square test (χ^2) measures the statistical significance of a difference in proportions and is the most commonly reported statistical test in the medical literature. It is the easiest statistical test to calculate manually (see the CAN'T MISS series supplement).

Example: (using the previously given appointment data): Fifteen of 30 men (50%) with appointments failed to keep them, whereas only 10 of 40 women (25%) failed to appear. The referent rate (RR) of missed appointments in men would be 0.5 ÷ 0.25 = 2 (i.e., men are twice as likely not to show up as women). While that may or may not fit the hypothesis about men's behavior in this situation, the statistical question is whether this 25% difference in the proportion of no-shows might have happened by chance sampling (in this case, scheduling might be causing the difference). The null hypothesis is that men and women fail to show up for appointments at about the same rate (i.e., RR = 1). Thus, χ^2 tests indicate the likelihood of noting a twofold difference in no-shows between the groups if in fact men and woman fail to keep their appointments at the same rate. The actual χ^2 value (test statistic) for these data is 5.84, which corresponds to a statistical significance *(p)* value of less than .02, meaning fewer than 2 out of every 100 days would result in a schedule where men were twice as likely not to show up. In other words, there is a 2% probability that the difference in no-shows by gender is due to chance, whereas there is a 98% probability the difference is due to some other factor or factors.

Table 1-5 summarizes the best types of statistical tests for healthcare studies. The list of Suggested Reading includes more detail on statistical analyses for quality improvement activities.

6. Concepts Related to Tests of Significance

a. Confidence Intervals

A *confidence interval* (CI) provides a range of possible values around a sample estimate (e.g., a mean, proportion, ratio) that is calculated from data. CIs commonly are used when comparing groups, but they also have other applications. They reflect the uncertainty that is always present when working with samples of subjects. The sample estimate(s) are a best guess about the true value of interest. For example, continuing the missed appointment example above, it is estimated that 50% of men miss their appointments, but the true value may be higher or lower. There is similar uncertainty about the true proportion of women who miss their appointments and about the ratio of the men's and women's proportions. Using the measure of variation from a sample, it is possible to construct a CI that, with a stated level of probability, holds the true value of interest.

Example: It was observed (hypothetically) that men are twice as likely to miss their appointments as women. The 95% CI around the RR of 2 is (1.27 – 3.13), meaning there is 95% certainty that men are between 0.27 and 3.13 times more likely to miss their appointment. A lower level of confidence would include a narrower range of values. For example, the 90% CI around the RR for the appointment data would be (1.44 – 2.77).

b. Level of Significance

The level of significance (*p*) gives the probability of observing a difference as large as the one found in a study when, in fact, there is no true difference between the groups (i.e., when the null hypothesis is true). A small *p* value indicates a small chance that the null hypothesis is true and favors the alternative hypothesis that there is a significance between the two groups. Historically, when the *p* value has been found to be less than .05, healthcare quality managers and researchers have declared their results statistically significant and "rejected the null hypothesis."

Example: The *p* value for the ratio of missed appointment rates above was .02, so it was concluded that there was little evidence that men and women had

Table 1-5. Statistics Reference Table

Independent Variable Groupings

Data Level/Intent	Nonparametric (Categorical/Nominal)	Parametric	
		Assumptions Violated or Ordinal Level Data	Assumptions Met
Inferential			
One-group	Chi-square goodness of fit (χ^2)		One-sample t test (t) Z approximation (1 sample z test)
Two-group-independent univariate	Chi-square	Kruskal-Wallis (H) Fishers exact test Mann Whitney (U)	One-way analysis of variance (ANOVA) (F) independent t test two-sample z test
Two-group paired univariate	McNemar test for significance of change	McNemar, Kappa Wilcox on matched pairs Signed rank test	Paired t test
More than two-group independent univariate	Chi-square	Kruskal-Wallis	ANOVA with post hoc analysis
More than two-group paired univariate	Cochran's Q		ANOVA with post hoc analysis
Repeated measures	Cochran's Q	Freidman test	Repeated measures ANOVA
Control for extraneous variables			Multivariate analysis of covariance (MANCOVA) ANCOVA
Multivariate analysis			Two-way or multivariate ANOVA
Association	Chi-square		Pearson's correlation (r)
Prediction			Regression modeling (F, r^2, R^2) Path analysis
Research summary/ synthesis			Meta-analysis (effect size)

the same rate of missed appointments ("the null") and determined that men probably had a higher rate of missed appointments. How much higher? There is 95% confidence that the true value lies between 0.27 and 3.13 times more likely to miss their appointments (see confidence interval example above). Note that if the p value had been >.05, the 95% CI would have been wider, determining that there was no difference in the proportions of men and women who miss their appointments.

G. Performance Improvement Tools

A variety of data analysis and graphic display tools are available to assist with understanding a process over time. Although no individual tool can support an entire process improvement team, tools can be used in combination to facilitate making data-based decisions. However, the use of tools alone does not guarantee accurate and effective decision making. Quality improvement teams must be configured to include frontline caregivers, key stakeholders across disciplines, and healthcare quality professionals with expertise in quality improvement design, implementation, and evaluation (including the tools and statistics described in this section). The management of data, analysis of information, and management through knowledge are necessary to change and improve healthcare organizations. For the tools to be successful, a strong team facilitator is necessary. There are many tools that are useful in the analysis of current processes and the design of new processes; this discussion is not meant to be all-inclusive. (Please refer to other reading materials for additional information and detail concerning tools available to healthcare quality professionals.)

Described next are performance improvement methods and tools for decision making, data analysis and process improvement, SPC, and measuring variation. Detailed descriptions and examples of these tools follow.

1. Decision-Making Methods and Tools

Brainstorming (Figure 1-5). *Brainstorming* is a free-flowing generation of ideas. This approach has the potential to generate excitement, equalize involvement, and result in original solutions to the problem. There is no censoring or discussion of ideas as they are generated, but the team can build upon the ideas of others. It is very important that no judgments are made concerning the idea's worth to the process, or whether the idea is even feasible (money is no object in a brainstorming exercise). Discussion of ideas comes at a later point in the process. This technique works well to generate ideas for tools including the cause-and-effect diagram and the tree diagram.

Figure 1-5. Brainstorming

Brainstorming is a free-flowing generation of ideas. This approach has the potential to generate excitement, equalize involvement, and result in original solutions to the problem. There is no censoring or discussion of ideas as they are generated, but the team can build upon the ideas of others. It is very important that no judgments are made concerning the idea's worth to the process, or whether the idea is even feasible (money is no object in a brainstorming exercise). Discussion of ideas comes at a later point in the process.

How to construct

1. Define the brainstorming topic.
2. Inform participants of the ground rules that (a) "all ideas are good ideas" and (b) "all comments/evaluation should be held in abeyance until the brainstorming is complete."
3. Give everyone a few minutes to think about the topic and to write down their ideas.
4. Have the team members call out their ideas. This can either be free-flowing, or a structure could be utilized such as going around the table with each person giving one idea each time around.
5. As the ideas are generated, one person should write the ideas on a flipchart.

When to use

- Use when a list of possible ideas is needed.
- This technique works well to generate ideas for such tools as the cause-and-effect diagram and the tree diagram, for example.

Multivoting (Figure 1-6). *Multivoting* is an easy, quick method for determining the most popular or important items from a list. This method utilizes a series of votes to cut the list in half each time, thus reducing the number of items to be considered.

Nominal group technique (Figure 1-7). This is a group decision-making process for generating a large number of ideas in which each member works by himself

Figure 1-6. Multivoting

Multivoting is an easy, quick method for determining the most popular or important items from a list. This method utilizes a series of votes to cut the list in half each time, thus reducing the number of items to be considered.

How to construct

1. Generate a list of items and number them.
2. If the group agrees, combine items that seem to be similar.
3. If necessary, renumber all items.
4. Each member lists on a sheet of paper the items s/he considers the most important (the number of items chosen should be at least one third of the total number of items on the list).
5. Tally the votes beside each item on the list.
6. Eliminate those items with the lowest scores.
7. Repeat the above process until the list is narrowed down to an appropriate number for the group to focus on or the item with the top priority is identified.

When to use

Use after a brainstorming session to identify the key items on which the group will focus.

Figure 1-7. Nominal Group Technique

This is a group decision-making process for generating a large number of ideas in which each member works by himself or herself. This technique is used when group members are new to each other or when they have different opinions and goals. This approach is more structured than that of brainstorming and multivoting.

How to construct

1. Define the task as you would for brainstorming.
2. Describe the purpose of this technique and the process to the group.
3. Write the question to be answered for all to see. Be sure to clarify the question as needed by the group.
4. Generate ideas to address the identified question by having the group write down their ideas in silence.
5. List all the items as you would in brainstorming, only be sure to use a structured approach so that all ideas are listed (again, there is to be no discussion of the items at this time).
6. Clarify and discuss the ideas one at a time.
7. Give each member from 4 to 8 cards or pieces of paper.
8. Members write one selection from the list on each card and assign a point value to each item. The highest value should be assigned to the most important item (i.e., if there are 4 cards, the most important card is numbered 4, next important 3, etc.)
9. The cards are collected and the votes are tallied; mark each item on the list with the value on the cards for that item.
10. The item with the largest number becomes the group's selection/priority.

When to use

- Use when the team members are new to each other.
- Use when dealing with a controversial topic.

or herself. This technique is used when group members are new to each other or when they have different opinions and goals. This approach is more structured than brainstorming and multivoting.

Delphi method (Figure 1-8). The Delphi method is a combination of the brainstorming, multivoting, and nominal group techniques. This technique is utilized when group members are not in one location and frequently is conducted by mail and or e-mail when a meeting is not feasible. After each step in the process, the data are sent to one person, who compiles the data and sends out the next round for participants to complete.

Figure 1-8. Delphi Method

The Delphi method is a combination of the brainstorming, multivoting, and nominal group techniques. This tool is utilized when the group is not in one location, such as in different offices around the country. The technique is frequently utilized through the mail and or e-mail when a meeting is not feasible. After each step in the process, the data are sent to one person who compiles the data and sends out the next step to the participants to complete.

Activity network diagram (Figure 1-9). This tool also is known as an arrow diagram (and in industry, it is also called a PERT [program evaluation and review technique] or a CPM [critical path method] chart). In the arrow diagram, the arrows connect articles (nodes) that represent a start and finish of activities. The arrows themselves represent the activities to be completed. Through the use of the arrow diagram, a sequence of events is depicted. It is useful when several simultaneous paths must be coordinated.

Figure 1-9. Activity Network Diagram

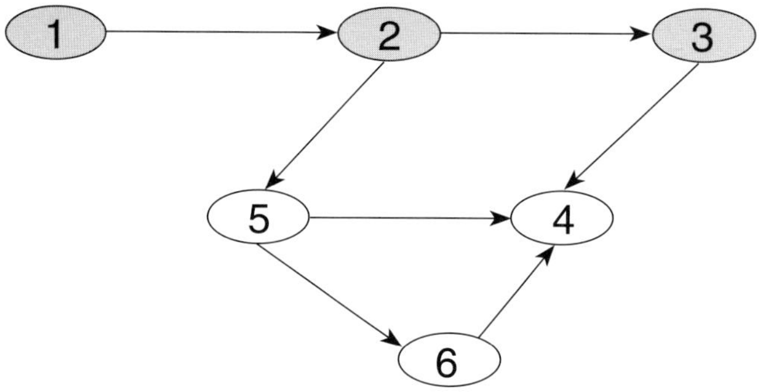

Another name for this tool is an arrow diagram and in industry, this tool is also called a PERT (program evaluation and review technique) or a CPM (critical path method) chart. In the arrow diagram, the arrows connect articles (nodes) that represent a start and finish of activities. The arrows actually represent the activities to be completed. Through the use of the arrow diagram, a sequence of events is depicted. It is useful when several simultaneous paths must be coordinated.

How to construct

1. List all the necessary tasks, one per card, to complete a project from start to finish.
2. Utilize the cards to sequence the activities for each path.
3. Identify the places in the paths where there are connections with other paths. These identify parts of one path that cannot be initiated until a point in another path is reached.
4. Determine the time duration for each task.
5. Calculate the shortest possible time to complete the project.
6. Review and revise the diagram as needed.

When to use

- Use when a task is complex and/or crucial to the organization.
- Use when simultaneous implementation of several paths must be coordinated.

Deployment chart (Figure 1-10). A deployment chart is used to project schedules for complex tasks and their associated subtasks. It usually is used with a task for which the time for completion is known. The tool also is used to determine who has responsibility for the parts of a plan or project. This tool also is called a *planning grid*. The grid helps the group organize the key steps in the project that will enable its members to reach the desired goal. Shaded boxes may be utilized to indicate who is primarily responsible, with ovals indicating an assistant or adviser.

Figure 1-10. Deployment Chart

	Bob	Linda	Roy	Sally	Tom
Chart Review at Hospital	X				
Chart Review at MD Office				X	
Interview Drs #123 and #456					X
Interview Office Nurses of Drs #123 and #456		X			
Compile Data			X		
Create Graphics			X		

A deployment chart is used to project schedules for complex tasks and their associated subtasks. It is usually used with a task for which the time for completion is known. The tool is also used to determine who has responsibility for the parts of a plan or project. Another name for this tool is a planning grid. The grid helps the group organize the key steps in the project that will enable its members to reach the desired goal. Shaded boxes may be utilized to indicate who is primarily responsible, with ovals indicating an assistant or adviser.

How to construct

1. Specify the outcome desired.
2. Identify the final step necessary (e.g., a report to a committee with the team's recommendations).
3. Identify the starting point.
4. Brainstorm a list of the necessary steps between the starting and final steps.
5. Refine the list by combining like steps and defining the sequence steps.
6. Design a grid with important items (e.g., who is responsible, due date, budget/cost) listed across the top.
7. Arrange the list of tasks or steps in sequence down the left column.
8. Fill in the appropriate columns, including tentative dates.
9. Revise the planning grid as necessary.

When to use

- Use as a planning tool to identify steps to be taken, timelines and responsibility for those steps.
- Use for project and management teams to determine what needs to be done, in what sequence, who is responsible for what, and how that relates to others.

Stratification chart (Figure 1-11). Stratification charts are designed to show where a problem does and does not occur, or to demonstrate underlying patterns. One such chart is called the Is/Is-Not Matrix. This matrix is used to organize knowledge and information so that patterns can be identified.

Histogram or bar chart (Figure 1-12). Before further analyzing a data set, the distribution of values for each of the variables should be reviewed. The optimal tool for reviewing a distribution depends on the amount of information. A bar graph with a separate bar for each value may be utilized when data are sparse (e.g., fewer than 12 values), but as the data increase, it becomes necessary to organize and summarize them.

A histogram, the most commonly used frequency distribution tool, does this by presenting the measurement scale of values along its x-axis (broken into equal-sized intervals) and the frequency scale (as counts or percents) along the y-axis.

Figure 1-11. Stratification Charts

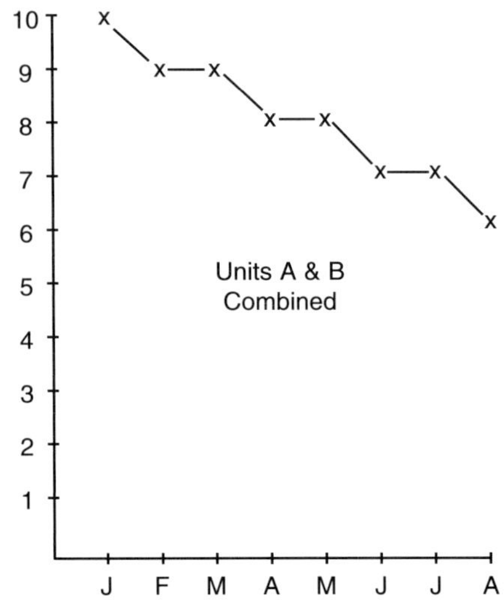

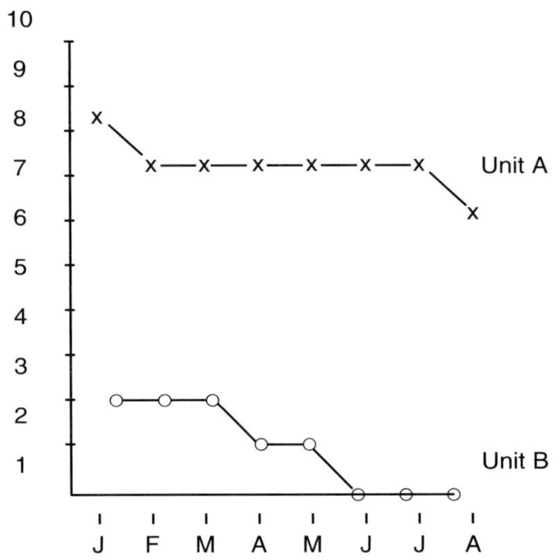

Stratification charts are designed to show where a problem does and does not occur, or to demonstrate underlying patterns. One such chart is called the Is/Is-Not Matrix. This matrix is used to organize your knowledge and information so that patterns can be identified.

How to construct

1. Examine the process to identify characteristics that could lead to biases and systematic differences in your results.
2. Enter data onto data collection forms (such as day of week or month, shifts or workers, etc.).
3. Look for patterns related to time and sequence.

Alternate tool: Is/Is-not Matrix

1. Enter data (such as where, when, what kind or how much, and who) onto a matrix in column on the left.
2. Across the top of the matrix list 3 columns: Is (when does something occur); Is Not (when does something not occur); and therefore (what might explain the pattern of occurrence).
3. Fill in the boxes.

When to use

- Use before data collection to know what difference or patterns to look for.
- Use after data collection to determine which factors actually affected the results.

Figure 1-12. Histogram or Bar Chart

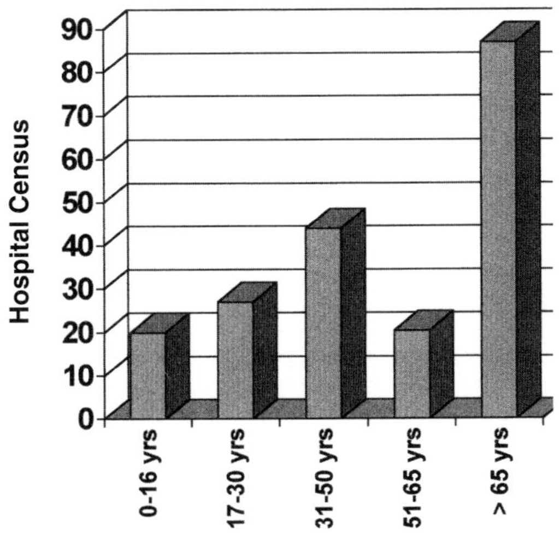

Before further analyzing a data set, one should first review the distribution of values for each of the variables. The optimal tool for reviewing a distribution depends on the amount of information. A bar graph with a separate bar for each value may be utilized when data are sparse (e.g., <12 values), but as the data increase, it becomes necessary to organize and summarize.

A histogram, the most commonly used frequency distribution tool, does this by presenting the measurement scale of values along its x-axis (broken into equal-sized intervals) and a frequency scale (as counts or percentages) along the y-axis. Plotting the frequency of each interval reveals the pattern of the data showing its center and spread (including outliers) and whether there is symmetry or skew. This is important information because it may reveal signals of problems in the data and should influence the choice of measure of central tendency and spread.

An important distinction must be made regarding bar charts and histograms. With a bar chart, the x-axis consists of discrete categories. Each bar is a separate group. An example of this would be plotting systolic blood pressure >140 by ethnic group. The height of the bar represents the frequency of the elevated blood pressure in each ethnic group. A histogram's x-axis is divided into categories using equally sized ranges of values along the axis. The variable is measured on a continuous scale, and therefore, the bars should not be separated by gaps between them. To continue with the systolic blood pressure example, the groupings of the 1-axis could be equal-sized with ranges defined as 90–99, 100–119, 120–129, etc. Histograms can be constructed manually or automatically via the use of various statistical software programs.

How to construct

1. Accumulate at least 25 data points (to give them least 5 bars).
2. Rank the data points from the smallest to the largest.
3. Calculate the range of the data by subtracting the smallest value from the largest.
4. Estimate the number of bars to be displayed (equals the square root of the number of data points).
5. Determine the width of the bars by dividing the range by the calculated number of bars, rounding the numbers as necessary.
6. Draw the vertical axis to show the number of times a value of the data falls with each bar.
7. Draw the horizontal axis to show the number of times a value of the data falls with each bar.
8. At the left side, draw bars with heights equal to the number of times the data fall within the bounds of each bar.
9. Label the histogram and describe the source, data and the author.

When to use

- Use to show the data's distribution or spread.
- Use to show whether the data are symmetric or skewed.
- Use to show whether there are extreme data values.

Plotting the frequency of each interval reveals the pattern of the data, showing their center and spread (including outliers) and whether there is symmetry or skew. This is important information because it may reveal problems in the data and should influence the choice of measure of central tendency and spread.

An important distinction must be made regarding bar charts and histograms. With a bar chart, the x-axis consists of discrete categories (each bar is a separate group). An example of this would be plotting systolic blood pressure >140 by ethnic group. The height of the bar represents the frequency of the elevated blood pressure for each 1 mm Hg change in each ethnic group. A histogram's x-axis is divided into categories using equally sized ranges of values along the axis. The variable is measured on a continuous scale, and therefore, the bars should not be separated by gaps. To continue with the systolic blood pressure example, the groupings of the 1-axis could be equal-sized, with ranges defined, for example, as 90–99, 100–119, 120–129 mm Hg. Histograms can be constructed manually or automatically with various statistical software programs.

Pareto diagram/Pareto chart (Figure 1-13). A Pareto diagram or chart displays a series of bars in which the priority for problem solving can easily be seen by the varying height of the bars. The tallest bar is the most frequently occurring issue. The bars are always arranged in descending height. This tool is related to the Pareto principle (named after the 19th century economist Vilfredo Pareto), which states that 80% of the problems or effects come from 20% of the causes. Therefore, by tackling 20% of the most frequent causes, an 80% improvement can be achieved.

Cause-and-effect, Ishikawa, or fishbone diagram (Figure 1-14). A cause-and-effect diagram is used to analyze and display the potential causes of a problem or the source of variation. There generally are at least four categories in the diagram. Some of the common categories include the four Ms: manpower, methods, machines, and materials; or the five Ps: patron (users of the system), people (workers), provisions (supplies), places to work (work environment), and procedures (methods and rules).

Scatter diagram or plot (Figure 1-15). A scatter diagram is used to determine the extent to which two variables (quality effects or process causes) relate to one another. These diagrams often are used in combination with fishbone or Pareto diagrams/charts. The extent to which the variables relate is called correlation. Scatter plots can be created manually or with statistical or spreadsheet software.

2. Data Analysis and Process Improvement

Failure mode and effects analysis (FMEA; Figure 1-16). FMEA is a preventive approach to identify failures and opportunities for error, and can be used for processes as well as equipment. The traditional techniques for FMEA originated in the manufacturing and other industries and have been adapted to healthcare. The Veterans Affairs National Center for Patient Safety has created HFMEA specifically for healthcare. There are six main steps to HFMEA™: (1) define a topic and process to be studied; (2) convene an interdisciplinary team with content and process experts; (3) develop a flow diagram of the process with consecutive numbering of each step and lettering of all subprocesses; (4) list all possible failure modes of each subprocess including the severity and probability of the failure mode, and then number these failure modes (brainstorming may be helpful to identify failure modes); (5) after analyzing the failure modes determine the action for each failure mode to eliminate, control, or accept and (6) identify the corresponding outcome measure to test the redesigned process (White, 2004).

Figure 1-13. Pareto Diagram or Chart

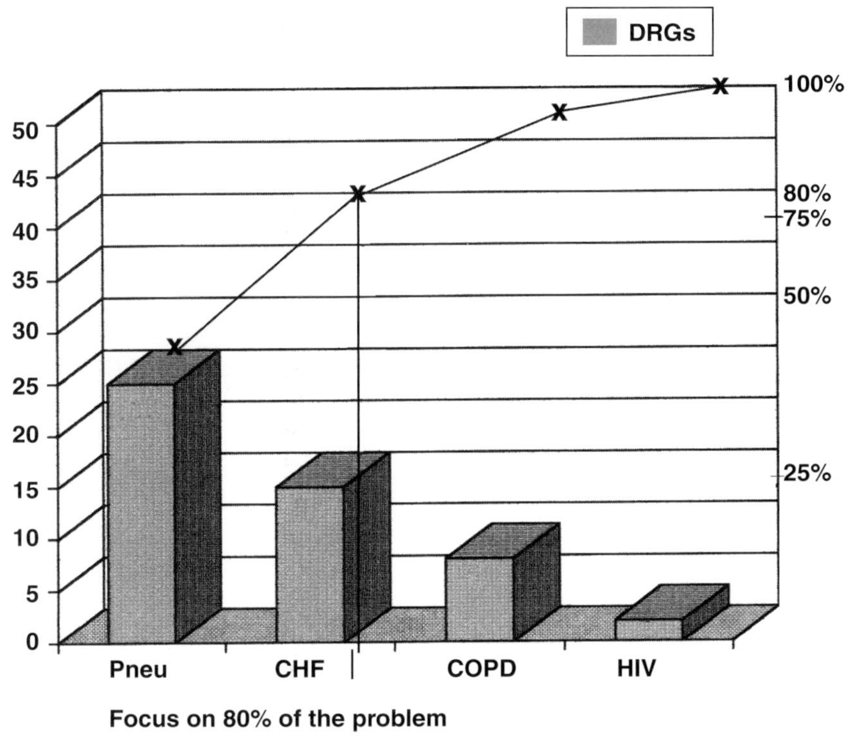

A Pareto diagram or chart displays a series of bars in which the priority for problem solving can easily be seen by the varying height of the bars. The tallest bar is the most frequently occurring issue. The bars are always arranged in descending height. This tool is related to the Pareto principle (named after the 19th century economist Vilfredo Pareto), which states that 80% of the problems or effects come from 20% of the causes. Therefore, by tackling 20% of the most frequent causes, an 80% improvement can be achieved.

How to construct

1. Identify the independent categories and the way to compare-either by frequency (count), time, cost, or other unity of analysis.
   Note: For 4 to 6 categories, have at least 30 data points. For 7 to 10 categories, have at least 60 data points. For 11 or more categories, have at least 100 data points.
2. Rank order the data in descending categories.
3. Calculate the percentage of the total each category depicts.

Thus far, the steps could be put into a table of data.

1. Draw the left, or vertical, axis with the unit of comparison.
2. Draw the horizontal axis with the categories, the largest to the smallest.
3. Draw a bar for each category.
4. Draw the right vertical axis from 0 to 100.
5. Draw a line graph of the cumulative percentage.
6. Label the axes and the diagram, noting the source of the data, the date, and the author.

When to use

To identify the most frequent or most important factors contributing to cost, problems, etc.

Figure 1-14. Cause-and-Effect Diagram or Ishikawa or Fishbone

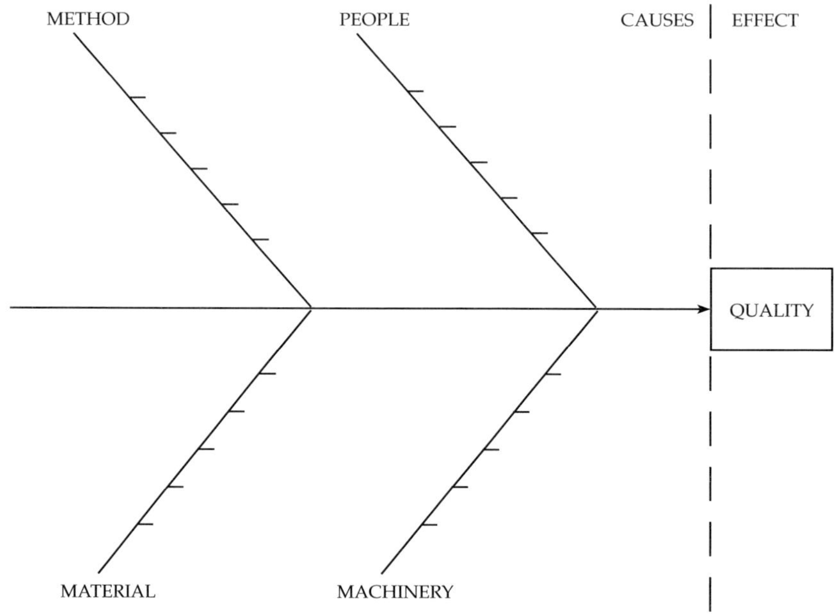

A cause-and-effect diagram is used to analyze and display the potential causes of a problem or the source of variation. There are generally at least four categories in the diagram. Some of the common categories include the four Ms—manpower, methods, machines and materials—or the five Ps—patron (users of the system), people (workers), provisions (supplies), places to work (work environment), and procedures (methods and rules).

How to construct

1. Determine the effect or the label for the diagram and put it on the far right side of the diagram.
2. Draw a horizontal line to the left of the effect.
3. Determine the categories (the four Ms or the five Ps).
4. Draw a diagonal line for half of the categories above the line and half the below the line.
5. Brainstorm the list for each of the categories.
6. Organize each of the causes on each bone.
7. Draw branch bones to show the relationships.

When to use

- To identify and organize possible causes of problems.
- To identify factors that will lead to success.
- As part of a root cause analysis.

Affinity diagram (Figure 1-17). The affinity diagram organizes numerous ideas or issues into groupings based on their natural relationships within the groupings. It typically is used to analyze or chart a process, and to structure and organize issues to provide a new perspective.

Interrelationship diagram (Figure 1-18). This tool organizes numerous complex problems, issues, or ideas by sorting and displaying their interrelations. This tool requires multidirectional thinking when there is not a straight-line cause-and-effect relationship. It is useful with both operational issues and organizational issues.

Figure 1-15. Scatter Diagram or Scatter Plot

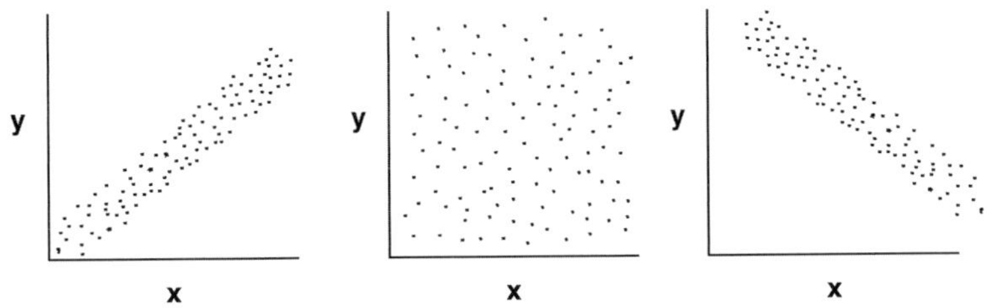

Positive Correlation
r->-o

No Correlation

Negative Correlation
r-<-o

A scatter diagram is used to determine the extent to which two variables, quality effects or process causes, relate to one another. These diagrams are often used in combination with Fishbone or Pareto Diagrams/Charts. The extent to which the variables relate is called correlation. Scatter plots can be created manually or with statistical or spreadsheet software.

How to construct

1. Collect at least 25 pairs of data for the two variables.
2. Draw and label the data over the equal distance on the graph.
3. Spread the data over equal distances on the graph.
4. Plot the paired sets of data by marketing the intersection of their values.
5. Label the scatter diagram and describe the source, date and the author.

When to use

- To determine whether there is a relationship between two variables.
- To determine the strength of the relationship-tight, loose, or outliers.
  Tight. The factors appear to be responsible for most of the variation.
  Loose. There are probably other factors affecting the data.
  Outliers. There are probably special causes present.
- To determine the type of relationship-positive, negative, or no relationship.
  Positive. As one variable increases, the other increases.
  Negative. As one variable increases, the other decreases.

Figure 1-16. Failure Mode and Effects Analysis (FMEA)

FMEA is a preventive approach to identify failures and opportunities for error. FMEA can be used for processes as well as equipment. The traditional techniques for FMEA been transferred from the manufacturing and other industries and has been adapted to healthcare.

The Veterans Affairs (VA) National Center for Patient Safety (http://www.patientsafety.gov/HFMEA.html) has created HFMEA™ specifically for healthcare.

How to construct

There are six main steps to HFMEA™:

1. Define a topic and process to be studied.
2. Convene an interdisciplinary team with content and process experts.
3. Develop a flow diagram of the process with consecutive numbering of each step and lettering of all sub-processes.
4. List all possible failure modes of each sub-process including the severity and probability of the failure mode and then number these failure modes (brainstorming may be helpful to identify failure modes).
5. After analyzing the failure modes determine the action for each failure mode to eliminate, control or accept.
6. Identify the corresponding outcome measure to test the redesigned process (White, 2004, p. 61).

Figure 1-17. Affinity Diagram

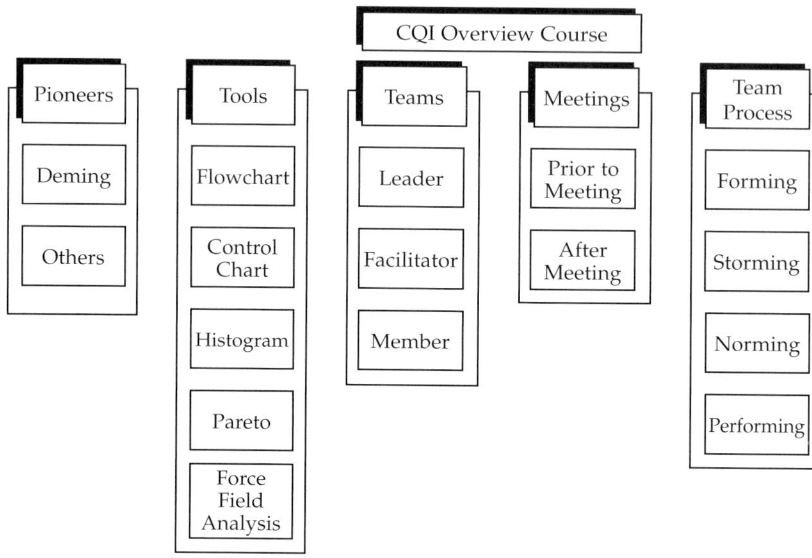

The affinity diagram organizes numerous ideas or issues into groupings based on their natural relationships within the groupings.

How to construct

1. Define the issue.
2. Brainstorm and record ideas on cards.
3. Randomly display the cards on a board.
4. Have the group silently sort the issues into groups.
5. Create header cards for grouping.
6. Draw a diagram based on the groupings (it will look like an organizational chart).

When to use

- To analyze or chart a process.
- To structure and organize issues to provide a new perspective.

Tree diagram (Figure 1-19). This tool maps out the full range of paths and tasks that are involved in the process and must be accomplished in order to achieve a goal. A tree diagram resembles an organizational chart. The tree diagram can be situated as an organizational chart or placed on its side.

Matrix diagram (Figure 1-20). This tool displays the connection between each idea or issue in one group to one or more groups. A matrix diagram can show the relationship between two items as well as the strength of the relationship. Many matrix diagram formats are available, but the L-shaped matrix is the most common. Other common formats include the T-shaped, Y-shaped, X-shaped, and the C-shaped matrices.

Prioritization matrix (Figure 1-21). This tool organizes tasks, issues, or actions and prioritizes them based on agreed-upon criteria. The tool combines the tree diagram and the L-shaped matrix diagram, displaying the best possible effect. The prioritization matrix often is utilized before more complex matrices are needed. This matrix applies options under discussion to the priority considerations of the organization.

Figure 1-18. Interrelationship Diagram

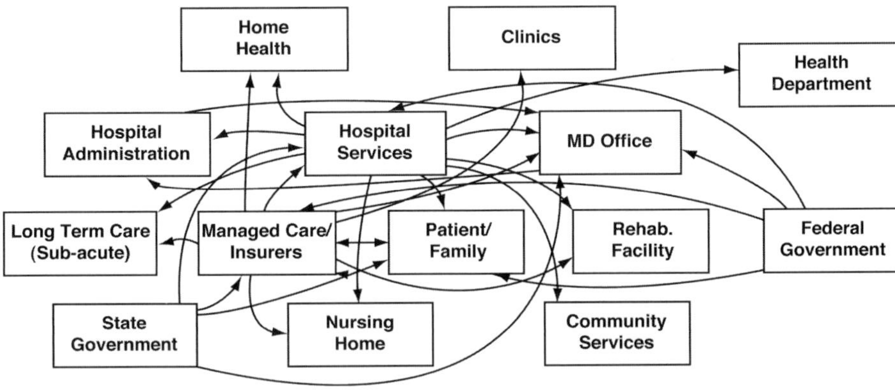

This tool organizes numerous complex problems, issues, or ideas by sorting and displaying their interrelations. This tool requires multidirectional thinking when there is not a straight-line cause-and-effect relationship. It is useful with both operational issues and organizational issues.

How to construct

1. Determine the issue/problem.
2. Generate ideas through brainstorming and other methods as to what the steps in the processes or issues might be.
3. Write the steps on cards and arrange them in similar groups (as with the affinity diagram), in cause-and-effect sequence. This technique is most effective when dealing with 15 to 50 items that may be interrelated. Discussion is appropriate throughout this process to ensure that no steps are missed.
4. Allow at least 1⁄2 inch of space between the cards to that relationship arrows can be drawn.
5. Fill in the relationship arrows that indicate what leads to what. This is done one card at a time until all cards have been discussed and relationship arrows drawn. Each card should be examined in terms of what happens when this card (process step) does occur; two-way arrows should be avoided.
6. Review and revise the diagram, transfer the information to a sheet of paper and distribute it to the team members for their review and revision prior to the next meeting.
7. Identify cards with the most arrows leading to them and cards with the most arrows leading away from the card (the cards with incoming arrows represent a secondary issue or bottleneck in a process; the cards with outgoing arrows indicate a basic cause/issue that, if solved or overcome, will affect a large number of other items); those cards with the most arrows leading away from the card (the cards with incoming arrows represent a secondary issue or bottleneck in a process; the cards with outgoing arrows indicate a basic cause/issue that, if solved or overcome, will affect a large number of other items); those cards with the greatest number of arrows are key factors in the process and should be addressed first.

When to use

- When the correct sequencing of events is critical.
- When the issue/problem is complex and contains interrelationships among and between ideas/steps.

Figure 1-19. Tree Diagram

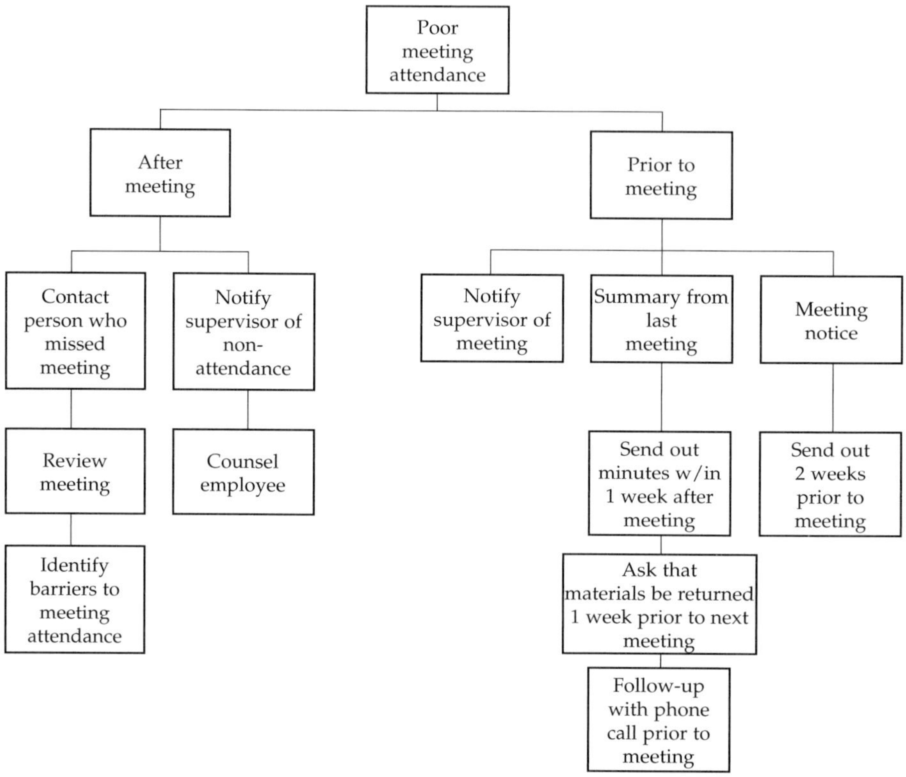

This tool maps out the full range of paths and tasks that are involved in the process and which must be accomplished in order to achieve a goal. A tree diagram resembles an organizational chart. The tree diagram can be situated as an organizational chart or placed on its side.

How to construct

1. Identify the overall goal that can be broken down into the steps necessary in order to achieve it.
2. Lay the paper you are working on vertically since the diagram is usually long rather than wide: work from left to right with the goal on the far left.
3. Select the appropriate tree branches (categories/groups) to investigate (an affinity diagram is often helpful to identify the first level of detail which is always the broadest level of detail); create headers for each of these branches.
4. For each header, ask: What needs to happen to achieve the header and thus goal statement? Write ideas on cards and place them to the right of the appropriate first level idea. This level should have a direct cause-and-effect relationship with the previous level.
5. When complete, ask the following questions to each level of detail: Will these actually lead to the results? Do we really need to do this task to reach the results?

When to use

- When it is crucial that a step/task not be overlooked.
- When a specific task has become the focus, but it is a complicated task to complete.
- When there have been numerous roadblocks to implementation.

Figure 1-20. Matrix Diagram

	Governing Body	Administrative Team	Medical Staff Leaders	Middle Management	Staff Members
Overview Course	▲	▲	▲	▲	▲
Team Training		■	■	■	●
Facilitator Training		■	■	■	●
Just-in-time Training		●	▲	▲	▲
Systems Thinking	▲	▲	▲	●	
Principle Centered Leadership	▲	▲	▲	●	

▲ Very important ■ Moderately important, as appropriate ● As needed

This tool displays the connection between each idea or issue in one group to one or more groups. A matrix diagram can show the relationship between two items as well as the strength of the relationship. Many matrix diagram formats are available to utilize, but the L-shaped matrix is the most common. Other common matrix formats include the T-shaped, Y-shaped, X-shaped, and the C-shaped matrices.

How to construct

1. Select the appropriate matrix format (e.g., L-shaped: 2 sets of items; T-shaped: 3 sets of items showing both indirect and direct relationships). Place the appropriate items on each axis of the matrix.
2. Determine the relationship symbols to be utilized (for example, the following symbols could be selected to indicate: # = strong relationships, * = some relationships, @ = weak/possible relationship).
3. Create the matrix and indicate the relationships.

When to use

- When defined tasks are to be assigned to employees.
- When comparing tasks to a set of criteria.
- When evaluating products or services against certain criteria.
- When determining the relationship between patient satisfaction and certain factors.

Flowchart or process flowchart (Figure 1-22). The *flowchart* or *process flowchart* is a graphical display of a process as it is known to its authors, owners, or team. The flowchart outlines the sequence and relationship of the pieces of the process. Through management of the data and information, the team comes to common understanding and knowledge concerning the process. Information is discussed about the structure (who carries out the specific step in the identified process), what activity is occurring, and the outcome or the results.

Process decision program chart (PDPC; Figure 1-23). This tool maps the identified events and contingencies that can occur from a problem statement to its solution. It attempts to identify potential deviations from the desired process, thus allowing the team to anticipate and prevent the deviation. PDPCs should be used when the team is uncertain about a proposed implementation plan. This tool can be displayed in a graphic format combining a tree diagram and a flowchart

Figure 1-21. Prioritization Matrix

	Low Cost	High Strategic Priority	Meets Accred. Standards	MD Concern	Staff Concern	Totals
Repair roof	3	4	2	3	4	16
Purchase new X-ray machine	5	2	0	1	5	13
Develop skilled nursing	4	1	0	2	2	9
Develop better commu-nications with home health	2	3	1	4	3	13
Develop a staff newsletter	1	5	3	5	1	15

This tool organizes tasks, issues, or actions and prioritizes them on agreed-upon-criteria. The tool combines the Tree Diagram (Figure 1-19) and the L-shaped Matrix Diagram (Figure 1-20), displaying the best possible effect. The prioritization matrix is often utilized before more complex matrices are needed. This matrix applies options under discussion to the priority considerations of the organization.

How to construct

1. Create a L-shaped matrix as previously described in the matrix section.
2. Prioritize and assign weights to the list of criteria that will be utilized in the prioritization.
3. Prioritize the list of options based upon each criterion.
4. Prioritize and select the item(s) across all of the criteria.

When to use

- When issues are identified and options must be narrowed down.
- When options have strong interrelationships.
- When options all need to be done, but prioritization or sequencing is needed.

or as an outline format (the outline format may be more difficult to use when communicating to a group and identifying patterns and simultaneous paths).

Run or trend chart (Figure 1-24). *Run* or *trend charts* are graphic displays of data points over time. Run charts are control charts without the control limits. Their name comes from the fact that the user is looking for trends in the data or a significant number of data points going in one direction or on one side of the average.

Trends generally indicate a statistically important event that needs further analysis. Resist the tendency to see every variation in the data as significant, by waiting to interpret the results until at least 10 (or even better, 20) data points have been plotted. As indicated in this example, it is best not to analyze data too frequently. For instance, looking at quarterly data may more accurately reflect trends over time than would reviewing data on a monthly basis.

Figure 1-22. Flowchart or Process Flowchart

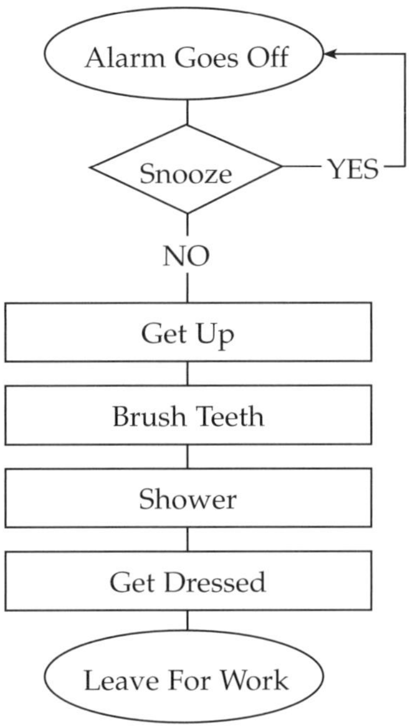

The flowchart or process flow chart is a graphical display of a process as it is known to its authors, owners, or team. The flowchart outlines the sequence and relationship of the pieces of the process. Through management of the data and information, the team comes to common understanding and knowledge concerning the process. Information is discussed on the structure (who carries out the specific step in the identified process), what activity is occurring, and the out-come or the results.

How to construct

1. Select the process to study.
2. Determine the beginning and the end or the boundaries of the process being studied.
3. The beginning or first step is put inside an oval symbol.
4. Each of the next steps is put in a rectangle.
5. When a step in the process involves a decision, the step is described in a diamond. A "yes" and a "no" path or line is drawn from the diamond.
6. Each decision loop reenters the process and is pursued to a conclusion.
7. The ending step, like the beginning step, is put inside an oval.

Other symbols include a triangle to describe step where storage or waiting occurs, an arrow to describe transport, and small circles with matching numbers to describe when a diagram must be continued in more then one page or column.

When to use

- To clarify a process.
- To reclarify a process revision.
- To describe a procedure.
- To identify internal and external customers.
- To identify potential areas of variability.

3. Statistical Process Control

Control chart (Figure 1-25). *Control charts* are run charts to which control limits have been added above and below the center line (mean). These lines are calculated from the data and show the range of variation in the output of a process. In general, upper and lower control limits (UCL and LCL) are determined by adding and subtracting three standard deviations to or from the mean. Assuming a normal distribution and no special cause variation, 99% of the data points would be expected to fall between the UCL and LCL.

There are many types of control charts for both variable and attributes data:

- variables data: 1 and range chart; median and range chart; *x* and *s* chart; *XmR* chart; moving average chart
- attributes data: P chart; NP chart; U chart; C chart.

One common chart presents the individual values (*X*) and calculates the limits based on the moving range (*mR*); this is the *XmR* chart. The *XmR* chart is used when data are obtained on a periodic basis, such as once a day or once a week, as is common in quality management activities.

Figure 1-23. Process Decision Program Chart (PDPC)

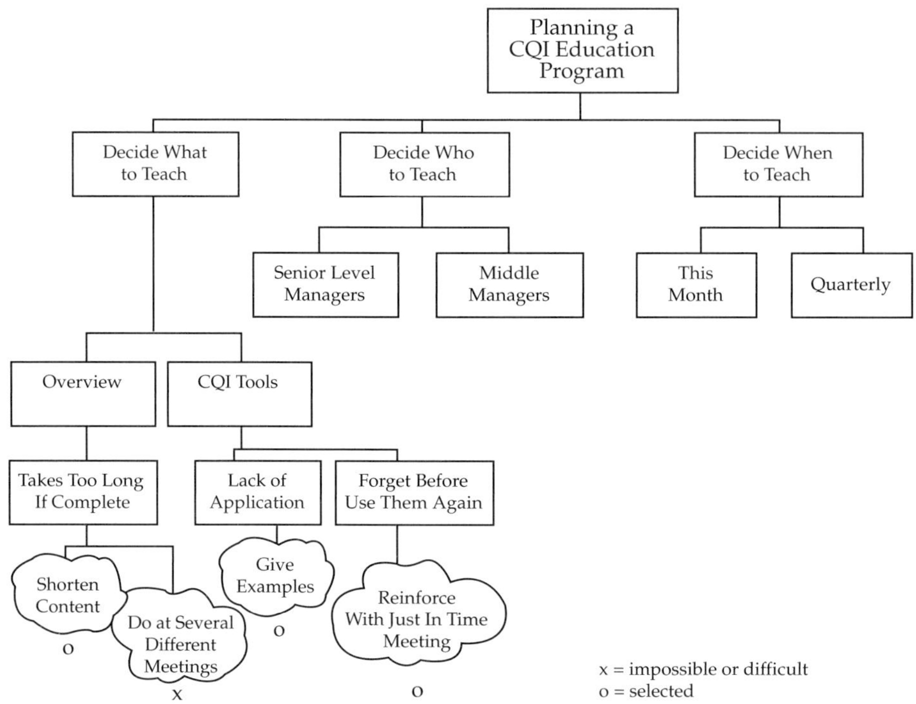

This tool maps out the identified events and contingencies that can occur from a problem statement to solution. This tool attempts to identify potential deviations from the desired process, thus allowing the team to anticipate and be proactive in prevention of the deviation. This tool should be utilized when the team is uncertain about a proposed implementation plan. This tool can be displayed in a graphic format combining a tree diagram and a flowchart, or it can be displayed as an outline format. The outline format may be more difficult to use when communicating to a group and identifying patterns and simultaneous paths.

How to construct

1. Determine the proposed flow of a process.
2. Choose the graphic or outline format.
3. Identify the desired goal or improvement.
4. List the first steps in sequence along the first level of the tree diagram, then add a second level of steps to reach the first-level steps (refer to how to construct a tree diagram for construction directions).
5. Identify what could go wrong at each step and list these as another level below the appropriate step.
6. Brainstorm ideas that could be implemented to prevent the undesired events and display them as clouds branched below the last level.

When to use

- As part of a root cause analysis.
- To anticipate any problems before implementing an action plan.
- To develop a contingency plan.
- To test theories as they are implemented if unable to test theory prior to implementation.

Figure 1-24. Run or Trend Chart

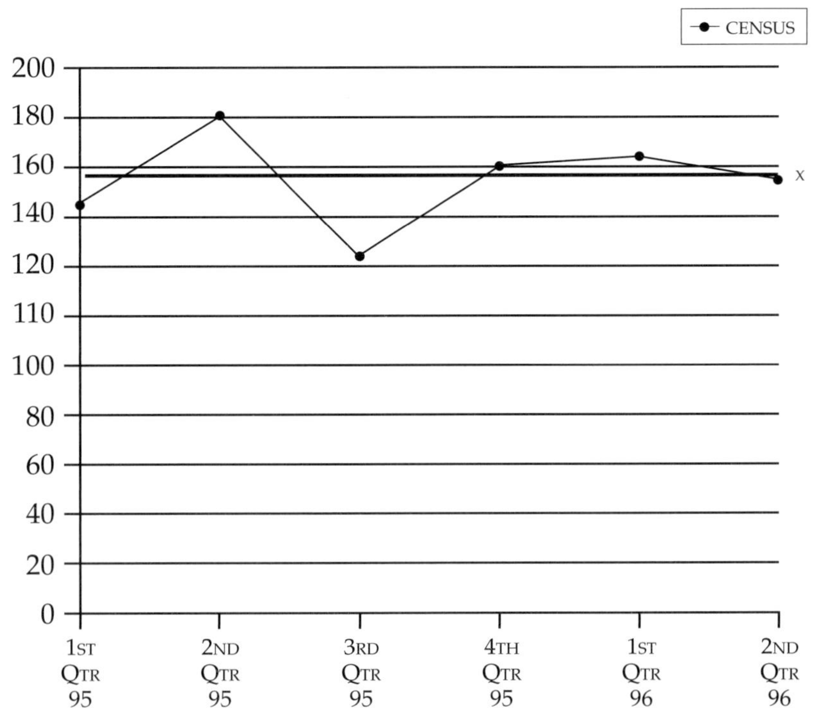

Run or trend charts are graphic displays of data points over time. Run charts are control charts without the control limits. Their name comes from the fact that the user is looking for trends in the data or significant number of data points going in one direction or on one side of the average.

Trends generally indicate a statistically important event that needs further analysis. Resist the tendency to see every variation in the data as significant by waiting to interpret the results until at least 10 (or even better, 20) data points have been plotted. As indicated in this example, it is best not to analyze data too frequently. For instance, looking at monthly data when quarterly data may more accurately reflect trends over time.

How to construct

1. Draw vertical and horizontal axes.
2. Label the vertical axis with the indicator or the variable and determine the scale.
3. Label the horizontal axis horizontal axis with the unit of time or sequence for which the data were collected.
4. Plot the data points.
5. Connect the data points.
6. Determine the mean of the plotted numbers and draw a mean line on the graph.
7. Label the chart and name the source of the data, date and the author.

When to use

- To display variation.
- To detect the presence or absence of special causes.
- To observe the effects of a process improvement (observe the effects of experiments on a process).

Figure 1-25. Control Chart

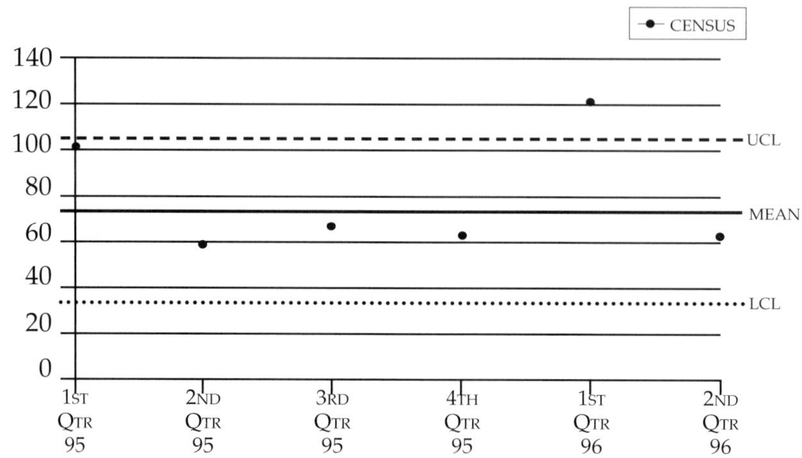

Control charts are run charts to which control limits have been added above and below the center line (mean). These lines are calculated from the data and show the range of variation in the output of a process. An example of a control chart is shown above.

Generally, upper and lower control limits (UCL and LCL) are statistically determined by adding and subtracting three standard deviations to or from the mean. Assuming a normal distribution, and no special cause variation, 99% of the data points would be expected to fall between the upper and lower control limits.

There are many type of control charts for both variable and attributes data. These include

- Variables data: 1 and range chart; median and range chart; x and s chart; XmR chart; moving average chart
- Attributes data: P chart; NP chart; U chart; and C chart.

One common chart presents the individual values (*X*) and calculates the limits based on the moving range (*mR*); this is the *XmR* chart. The *XmR* chart is used when data are obtained on a periodic basis, such as once a day or once a week, as is common in quality management activities.

How to construct

1. Construct chart as you would a run or trend chart.
2. Calculate control limits according to the appropriate statistical formula or via computer program.
3. Plot the control limits on the chart and examine the data for variation as described below.

When to use

- To distinguish variation from common and special causes.
- To assist with eliminating special cause variation.
- To observe effects of a process improvement.

4. Types of Variation

Common cause variation. Variation is inherent in any process. On a control chart, this type of variation is exhibited as points between the control limits in no particular pattern. This is variation that normally would be expected from a process. If this type of variation is treated as being unpredictable, it could tamper with the process and, in fact, make things worse. The root cause of the variation must be identified prior to trying to "fix" the problem.

Special cause variation. Variation that arises from sources that are not inherent in the process are unpredictable. On a control chart, this type of variation is exhibited as points that fall outside the control limits; or, when inside the control limits, exhibit certain patterns. These special cause variations should be addressed any time that they occur with interventions appropriate for the elimination of the special cause, if possible.

Root cause analysis. When variation is inherent in the process and a reduction of the variation is desired, the root cause of the variation must be identified to eliminate tampering with the effective components of the process. This is a requirement of the Joint Commission in response to sentinel events. To start with, potential causes of the variation should be identified. An interdisciplinary team very familiar with the process should utilize brainstorming, flowcharting, and/or cause-and-effect diagrams or some other process to determine these potential causes. The second step is to verify the potential causes by collecting data concerning the process. After the data are collected and analyzed utilizing the tools discussed in this module, the actual causes of the variation (or at least the most probable causes) can be identified. The following areas should be addressed in the analysis:

- human factors—communications and information management systems
- human factors—training
- human factors—fatigue/scheduling
- environment factors
- equipment factors
- rules, policies, procedures
- leadership systems and culture (White, 2004).

At this point, the team should develop and implement an action plan designed to eliminate or minimize the root cause(s) of the variation.

Figure 1-26. Force Field Analysis

CQI Education Program

STRENGTHS	BARRIERS
Management supports program →	← Lack of time
Physicians support program →	← Lack of commitment of all participants
Have committed time and other resources to complete program →	← Viewed as not important

Force field analysis is a method to systematically identify the various forces that facilitate or increase the likelihood of success, and the opposite factors, those that decrease or restrain the likelihood of success or improvement in the process. This chart is similar to listing the pros and cons of an action.

How to construct

1. Identify the issue.
2. Create two columns on a sheet of paper. Label one "strengths" and one "barriers."
3. Brainstorm and list potential strengths and barriers on the chart.
4. Determine actions to be taken to increase the strengths and to decrease or eliminate the barriers.

When to use

To identify the strengths of barriers for the success of a project.

Force field analysis (Figure 1-26). *Force field analysis* is a method to systematically identify the various forces that facilitate or increase the likelihood of success, and the opposite factors, those that decrease or restrain the likelihood of success or improvement in the process. This chart is similar to listing the pros and cons of an action.

Frequency distribution (Figure 1-27). Bell curves, histograms, and 2 x 2 tables are all types of *frequency distributions*. When people describe a normal distribution, they are referring to a bell curve. Displaying the frequency distribution can help determine if one or more processes are occurring. For example, a frequency distribution can be a bimodal distribution of the ages of patients undergoing a total hip replacement. In other words, the data essentially have two different bell curves present, and possibly two different processes. Conceivably, the demographics and risk factors may be different, and each age distribution may need a separate quality improvement focus.

Figure 1-27. Frequency Distribution

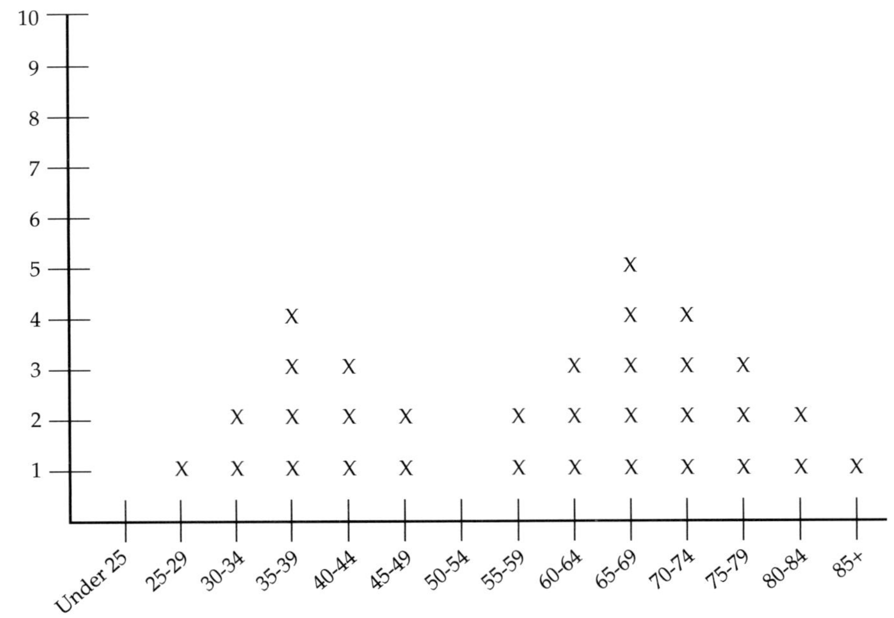

Bell curves, histograms, and 2 x 2 tables are all types of frequency distributions. When people describe a normal distribution, they are referring to a bell curve. Displaying the frequency distribution can help determine if one or more processes are occurring. For example, a frequency distribution can be a bimodal distribution of the ages of patients undergoing a total hip replacement. In other words, the data essentially have two different bell curves present, and possibly two different processes. Conceivably, the demographics and risk factors may be different, and each age distribution may need a separate quality improvement focus.

How to construct

1. Develop a scale based on the range of data to be collected.
2. Count the data and mark the appropriate spot on the scale.

When to use

- When the spread or distribution of the data are important.
- When it is suspected that more than one process is going on.

References

Bader, B.S., & Bohr, D. (1991). *Guide to the interpretation and use of quality of care data*. Chicago: American Hospital Association, The Hospital Research and Education Trust.

Barry R., Murcko, A.C., & Brubaker, C.E. (2002). *The six sigma book for healthcare*. Chicago: Health Administration Press.

Batalden, P.B., & Buchanan, E.D. (1989). Industrial models of quality improvement. In N. Goldfield & D. Nash (Eds.), *Providing quality care*. (pp. 133–159). Philadelphia: American College of Physicians.

Bates, D.W., & Gawande, A.A. (2003). Improving safety with information technology. *New England Journal of Medicine, 348*, 2526–2534.

Becher, E.C., & Chassin, M.R. (2001). Improving the quality of healthcare: Who will lead? *Health Affairs, 20*, 164–179.

Berwick, D.M. (1989). Continuous improvement as an ideal in health care. *New England Journal of Medicine, 320*, 53–56.

Berwick, D.M., Godfrey, A.B., & Roessner, J. (1990). *Curing health care*. San Francisco: Jossey-Bass Publishers.

Blendon, R.J., DesRoches, C.M., Brodie, M., Benson, J.M., Rosen, A.B., Schneider, E., et al. (2002). Views of practicing physicians and the public on medical errors. *New England Journal of Medicine, 347*(24), 1933–1940.

Brassard, M. (1988). *The memory jogger*. Methuen, MA: Goal/QPC.

Burke, D., Menachemi, N., & Brooks, R.G. (2005). Diffusion of information technology supporting the Institute of Medicine's quality chasm care aims. *Journal for Healthcare Quality, 27*(1), 24–32.

Burton, W.N., & Hoy, D.A. (1993). First Chicago's integrated health data management computer system. *Managed Care Quarterly, 1*(3), 18–23.

Byers, J.F., & Beaudin, C.L. (2001). Critical appraisal tools facilitate the work of the quality professional. *Journal for Healthcare Quality, 23*(5), 35–38, 40–43.

Byers, J.F., & Beaudin, C.L. (2002). The relationship between continuous quality improvement and research. *Journal for Healthcare Quality, 24*(1), 4–8.

Byers J.F. & White S.V. (Eds.). *Patient safety: Principles and practice* (pp. 87–134). New York: Springer.

Chassin, M.R. (1998). Is health care ready for six sigma quality? *The Milbank Quarterly, 76*(4), 565–591. Retrieved April 5, 2005, from http://www.milbank.org/quarterly/764featchas.html

Codman, E.A. (1916 & 1972). *A study of hospital efficiency*. Ann Arbor, MI: University Microfilms.

Committee on Quality of Health Care in America (CQHCA), Institute of Medicine. (2000). *To err is human: Building a safer health system*. (L.T. Kohn, J.M. Corrigan, & M.S. Donaldson, Eds.) Washington, DC: National Academies Press. Also available online at www.nap.edu

Committee on Quality of Health Care in America (CQHCA), Institute of Medicine. (2001). *Crossing the quality chasm: A new health system for the 21st century*. Washington, DC: National Academies Press. Also available online at www.nap.edu

Crosby, P.B. (1979). *Quality is free: The art of making quality certain*. New York: McGraw-Hill.

Deaton, C. (2001). Outcomes measurement and evidence-based nursing practice. *Journal of Cardiovascular Nursing, 15*(2), 83–86.

de Brantes, F. (2003). Guest editorial: Bridges to excellence: A program to start closing the quality chasm in healthcare. *Journal for Healthcare Quality, 25*(2), 2, 11.

Deming, W.E. (2000a). *The new economics for industry, government, education*. Cambridge, MA: MIT Center for Advanced Engineering Studies.

Deming, W.E. (2000b). *Out of the crisis*. Cambridge, MA: MIT Center for Advanced Engineering Studies.

Donabedian, A. (1980). *Exploration in quality assessment and monitoring*. Ann Arbor, MI: Health Administration Press.

Gaucher, E.M., & Coffey, R.J. (1991). *Transforming healthcare organizations: How to achieve and sustain organizational excellence.* San Francisco: Jossey-Bass Publishers.

Greenhalgh, T. (1999). Narrative based medicine in an evidence-based world. *British Medical Journal, 318,* 323–325.

Harry, M., & Schroeder, R. (2000). *Six sigma: The breakthrough strategy revolutionizing the world's top corporations.* New York: Currency/Doubleday.

Hunt, V.D. (1992). *Quality in America: How to implement a competitive quality program.* Homewood, IL: Business One Irwin.

Integrated Healthcare Association. (2005). California leadership group of health plans, physician groups, and health systems. Available at http://www.iha.org.

James, B.C. (1990). *Quality management for health care delivery.* Chicago: The Hospital Research and Education Trust.

Joint Commission on Accreditation of Healthcare Organizations. (2004). *Crosswalk of 2003 patient rights and organization ethics for hospitals to 2004 ethics, rights and responsibilities for hospitals.* Retrieved June 10, 2004, from http://www.jcaho.org/accredited+organizations/hospitals/standards/new+standards/ri_xwalk_hap.pdf

Joint Commission on Accreditation of Healthcare Organizations. *Alternatives for sharing sentinel event related information with the Joint Commission.* Retrieved May 1, 2005 from http://www.jcaho.org/accredited+organizations/sentinel+event/reporting+alternatives.htm

Jones, D., & Womack, J. (2003). *Lean thinking: Banish waste and create wealth in your corporation, revised and updated.* New York: Free Press.

Juran, J.M. (1967, January). The QC circle phenomenon. *Industrial Control, 23,* 329–336.

Juran, J.M. (1977). *Quality and its assurance: An overview.* Presented at the Second NATO Symposium on Quality and Its Assurance, London.

Juran, J.M. (1981, June and July). Product quality: A prescription for the west. *The Management Review.* (First presented at the 25th Conference of the European Organization for Quality Control, Paris.)

Martin, K. (2003). On lean enterprise and its potential healthcare applications [Editorial]. *Journal for Healthcare Quality, 25*(5), 2, 43.

Merry, M. (1992). The evolution of quality assurance and an overview of total quality management. In J. Lord (Ed.), *The physician leader's guide.* Rockville, MD: Bader and Associates, Inc.

National Association for Healthcare Quality (NAHQ). (2004). *NAHQ Code of ethics and standards of practice for healthcare quality professionals.* Glenview, IL: Author. Retrieved April 5, 2005, from www.nahq.org/about/code.htm

National Committee for Quality Assurance. (2005). *HEDIS 2005,* Volumes 1 and 2. Washington, DC: Author.

National Committee on Vital and Health Statistics. (2002, February 27). *Letter to the Secretary: Recommendations for the first set of PMRI standards.* Washington, DC: Author. Retrieved April 5, 2005, from http://www.ncvhs.hhs.gov/020227lt.htm

O'Rourke, L.M., & Bader, B.S. (1993). An illustrative quality and performance report for the governing board. *The Quality Letter for Healthcare Leaders, 5*(2), 15–28.

Pelletier, L. R. (2000). On error-free healthcare: Mission possible! [Editorial]. *Journal for Healthcare Quality, 22*(3), 2.

Plsek, P., & Omnias, A. (1989). *Juran Institute quality improvement tools: Problem solving/glossary.* Wilton, CT: Juran Institute, Inc.

President's Information Technology Advisory Committee. (2004). *Health Care Delivery and Information Technology Subcommittee: Draft recommendations,* April 13, 2004. Retrieved April 5, 2005, from http://www.nitrd.gov/pitac

Quality Measurement and Management Project. (1991). *Hospital quality-related data: Recommendations for appropriate data requests, analysis, and utilization.* Chicago: American Hospital Association.

Revere, L., & Black, K., (2003). Integrating Six Sigma with total quality management: A case example for measuring medication errors. *Journal of Healthcare Management, 48*(6), 377–391.

Roberts, J.S., Redman, R.R., & Coate, J.G. (1987). A history of the Joint Commission on Accreditation of Hospitals. *The Journal of the American Medical Association, 258*, 936–940.

Rontal, R. (1993). Information and decision support in managed care. *Managed Care Quarterly, 1*(3), 3–14.

Rosati, R.J. (2003). Creating quality improvement projects. In E.L. Siegler, S. Mirafzali, & J.B. Foust (Eds.), *A guide to hospitals and inpatient care* (pp. 326–338). New York: Springer.

Sackett, D., Rosenberg, W. M.C., Muir-Gray, J.A., Haynes, R.B., & Richardson, W.S. (1996). Evidence-based medicine: What it is and what it isn't. *British Medical Journal, 312*(13), 71–72.

Tonelli, M. (2001). The limits of evidence-based medicine. *Respiratory Care, 46*(12), 1435–1440.

Tweed-Weber, Inc. (1992). *Total quality management in home health care*. Reading, PA: Author.

U.S. CFR parts 160 and 164. (Aug. 14, 2002). Standards for privacy of individually identifiable health information: final rule. *Federal Register*. Retrieved April 29, 2005, from http://www.hipaadvisory.com/regs/regs_in_PDF/finalprivmod.pdf

Versel, N. (March 29, 2005). Docs fight UH's pay-for-performance program. *Health-It World.* Available at http://www.health-itworld.com/enews/03-29-2005_557.html

Weiner, M., Callahan, C.M., Tierney, W.M., Overhage, J.M., Mamlin, B., Dexter, P.R., et al. (2003). Using information technology to improve health care of older adults, *Annals of Internal Medicine, 139*, 430–436.

Young, T., Brailsford, S., Connell, C., Davies, R., Harper, P., & Klein, J.H. (2004). Using industrial processes to improve patient care. *British Medical Journal, 328*, 162–164.

Suggested Reading

Anderson, S., & Wittwer, W. (2004). Using bar-code point-of-care technology for patient safety. *Journal for Healthcare Quality, 26*(6), 5–11.

Bakken, S., & Hripcsak, G. (2004). An informatics infrastructure for patient safety and evidence-based practice in home healthcare. *Journal for Healthcare Quality, 26*(3), 24–30.

Byers, J.F., & Aragon, E.D. (2003). What quality improvement professionals need to know about IRBs. *Journal for Healthcare Quality, 25*(4), 4–9.

Carter, K.J., Castro, F., Kessler, E., & Erickson, B. (2004). Simulation of breast cancer screening: Quality assessment of two protocols. *Journal for Healthcare Quality, 26*(6), 25–32.

Degnan, D., Merryfield, D., & Hultgren, S. (2004). Reaching out to clinicians: Implementation of a computerized alert system. *Journal for Healthcare Quality, 26*(6), 20–24.

Drain, M., & Clark, P.A. (2004). Measuring experience from the patient's perspective: Implications for national initiatives. *Journal for Healthcare Quality Online, 26*(4). Retrieved May 9, 2005, from http://www.nahq.org/journal/ce/article.html?article_id=215

Fortinsky, R.H., & Madigan, E. (2004). Data, information, and quality indicators for home healthcare: Rapid implementation, what's next? *Journal for Healthcare Quality, 26*(3), 44–51.

Genovich-Richards, J. (2003). Interview with a quality leader: Dale Schumacher on strategic quality planning and research. *Journal for Healthcare Quality, 25*(4), 16–18, 39.

Hamilton, E., Platt, R., Gauthier, R., McNamara, H., Miner, L., Rothenberg, S. et al. (2004). The effect of computer-assisted evaluation of labor on cesarean rates. *Journal for Healthcare Quality, 26*(1), 37–44.

Hansen, J.P. (2003a). CAN'T MISS—Conquer any number task by making important statistics simple. Part 1. Types of variables, mean, median, variance, and standard deviation. *Journal for Healthcare Quality, 25*(4), 19–24.

Hansen, J.P. (2003b). CAN'T MISS—Conquer any number task by making important statistics simple. Part 2. Probability, populations, samples, and normal distributions. *Journal for Healthcare Quality, 25*(4), 25–33.

Hansen, J.P. (2003c). CAN'T MISS—Conquer any number task by making important statistics simple. Part 3. Standard error, estimation, and confidence intervals. *Journal for Healthcare Quality, 25*(4), 34–39.

Hansen, J.P. (2004a). CAN'T MISS—Conquer any number task by making important statistics simple. Part 4. Confidence intervals with *t* distributions, standard error, and confidence intervals for proportions. *Journal for Healthcare Quality*, *26*(4), 26–32.

Hansen, J.P. (2004b). CAN'T MISS—Conquer any number task by making important statistics simple. Part 5. Comparing two confidence intervals, standard error of the difference between two means and between two proportions. *Journal for Healthcare Quality*, *26*(4), 33–42.

Hansen, J.P. (2004c). CAN'T MISS—Conquer any number task by making important statistics simple. Pary 6. Tests of statistical significance (*z* test statistic, rejecting the null hypothesis, *p* value), *t* test, *z* test for proportions, statistical significance versus meaningful difference. *Journal for Healthcare Quality*, *26*(4), 43–53.

Hansen, J.P. (2005a). CAN'T MISS: Conquer any number task by making important statistics simple. Part 7. Statistical process control: $\bar{x}$–*s* control charts. *Journal for Healthcare Quality*, *27*(4), 32–43.

Hansen, J.P. (2005b). CAN'T MISS: Conquer any number task by making important statistics simple. Part 8. Statistical process control: *n, np, c, u* control charts. *Journal for Healthcare Quality*, *27*(4), 45–52.

Lathrop, C.B. (2003). Setting up QI programs for pediatric specialty clinics. *Journal for Healthcare Quality*, *25*(6), 10–16, 27.

Maese, J.R. (2003). Demonstrating clinical oversight and effectiveness in the ambulatory setting—An ambulatory report card. *Journal for Healthcare Quality*, *25*(2), 38–45.

Mears, D. (2004). Interview with a quality leader: Scott Wallace on information technology and advancing healthcare quality. *Journal for Healthcare Quality*, *26*(6), 17–19.

Menachemi, N., Burke, D., & Brooks, R. (2004). Adoption factors associated with patient safety-related information technology. *Journal for Healthcare Quality*, *26*(6), 33–38.

Miceli, P.J. (2004). Validating a patient satisfaction survey translated into Spanish. *Journal for Healthcare Quality*, *26*(4), 4–13.

Orton, J.A., Jacobson, J., & Haug, P (2003). Automation of performance measures reporting. *Journal for Healthcare Quality*, *25*(5), 21–27.

Polizzi, J., Byers, J.F., & Kiehl, E. (2003). Co-bedding versus traditional bedding of multiple-gestation infants in the NICU. *Journal for Healthcare Quality*, *25*(1), 5–11.

Rao, N., Schilling, D., Rice, J., Ridenour, M., Mook, W., & Santa, E. (2004). Prevention of postoperative mediastinitis: A clinical process improvement model. *Journal for Healthcare Quality*, *26*(1), 22–28, 60.

Sevcik, A.E., Abu-Jaber, T., & Marek, L. (2004). Understanding approaches to case-mix assessment and case-mix adjustment. *Journal for Healthcare Quality Online*, *26*(5). Retrieved May 9, 2005, from http://www.nahq.org/journal/online/sep_oct/Understanding_Approaches.pdf

Soroka, M., Feldman, L., & Crump, T. (2004). Quality-of-care review of optometric records: Inter-rater reliability. *Journal for Healthcare Quality*, *26*(5), 29–33.

White, S.V. (2003). Second Annual Summit on Patient Safety and Information Technology. *Journal for Healthcare Quality*, *25*(6), 38–39, 45.

White, S.V. (2004). Interview with a quality leader: David Brailer on information technology and advancing healthcare quality. *Journal for Healthcare Quality*, *26*(6), 20–25.

MODULE TWO

Strategy and Leadership

Jean Grube, PhD MBA MSN

MODULE TWO

I. Introduction

Total quality management (TQM) is "a strategic, integrated management system, which involves all managers and employees and uses quantitative methods to continuously improve an organization's processes to meet and exceed customer needs, wants, and expectations" (Stamatis, 1996, p. 58). In recent years, customers have increasingly scrutinized the U.S. healthcare system and the results of the examination are not favorable. In response to the public's concern, the Institute of Medicine (IOM) identified six aims for healthcare improvement:

- *Safety*—avoiding injuries to patients from care that is intended to help them
- *Effectiveness*—providing services based on scientific knowledge to all who could benefit, and refraining from providing services to those not likely to benefit (avoiding overuse and underuse)
- *Patient-centeredness*—providing care that is respectful of and responsive to individual patient preferences, needs, and values, and ensuring that patient values guide all clinical decisions
- *Timeliness*—reducing waits and sometimes harmful delays for both those who receive and those who give care
- *Efficiency*—avoiding waste, in particular waste of equipment, supplies, ideas, and energy
- *Equity*—providing care that does not vary in quality with respect to personal characteristics, ethnicity, geographic location, or socioeconomic status (Committee on Quality of Health Care in America [CQHCA], 2001, p. 6).

This module addresses the role of strategic management and leadership in reaching those aims. To navigate these complex issues, some type of framework or roadmap is required. The framework used in this module views healthcare organizations as complex systems.

II. Healthcare Organizations as Complex Systems

A. Definition and Importance

The primary dictionary definition of *system* is, "a regularly interacting or interdependent group of items forming a unified whole" (Merriam-Webster's Collegiate Dictionary, 1994, p. 1197). The value of having a systems perspective is that "systems thinking" is a discipline for seeing wholes. It is a framework for seeing interrelationships, rather than things; for seeing patterns of change rather than static "snapshots" (Senge, 1990). "Today, systems thinking is needed more than ever because we are becoming overwhelmed by complexity" (Senge, p. 69). Benefits of systems thinking include

- aiding in identifying and understanding the "big picture"
- facilitating the identification of major components
- identifying important relationships and providing proper perspective
- avoiding excessive attention to a single part
- allowing for a broad scope solution
- fostering integration
- providing a basis for redesign (Ginter, Swayne, & Duncan, 2002).

Viewing organizations as complex systems is consistent with the principles of quality pioneers such as Deming (1986) and Juran (1989), as TQM practices influence all processes, functions, and departments within an organization. Making changes in one process or department naturally will require changes in other processes, functions, and departments. Thus, effectiveness is dependent on alignment of the parts of the system.

Healthcare organizations are among the most complex entities, with ever-changing technology, new environmental pressures on nearly a daily basis, and complicated relationships among professionals, disciplines, departments, and organizations. Hence, research suggests that healthcare leaders must consider the science of complex adaptive systems (CAS) in order to effectively manage and improve their organizations. *Complex* implies diversity—a wide variety of elements. *Adaptive* suggests the capacity to alter or change—the ability to learn from experience. A *system* is a set of connected or interdependent things (Begun, Zimmerman, & Dooley, 2003).

Table 2-1 depicts the tasks that leadership must assume as they move from a classic (bureaucratic) organization to one that has the characteristics of CAS.

Table 2-1. Leadership Tasks in Classic Design and Complex Adaptive Systems

Classic Design/Bureaucracy	Complex Adaptive System
• Role-defining	• Relationship-building
• Tight-structuring	• Loose-coupling
• Simplifying	• Complicating/linking
• Socializing	• Diversifying
• Decision-making	• Sense-making
• Planning based on forecasting	• Thinking about the future
• Controlling	• Improvising
• Knowing	• Learning

Source: Anderson & McDaniel, 2000.

B. Frameworks for Studying Healthcare Systems

A variety of systems models exist. "The model that the manager selects is less important than how he or she uses it to begin recognizing, understanding, and anticipating how the parts of the systems interact as a whole" (Kelly, 2003, p. 73).

Avedis Donabedian is credited as being the founder of the quality assurance field. As a researcher and physician at the University of Michigan, he developed a theoretical framework for patient care evaluation (Donabedian, 1980). The model describes the importance of relating healthcare structures and processes to how clients actually fared because of their care. *Structures* are the resources available for care delivery, whereas *processes* involve the care (how patients were diagnosed and treated). Outcomes include the results of that care (e.g., satisfaction, length and quality of life; see **Figure 2-1**).

Figure 2-1. Donabedian's Framework

Structure	Process	Outcomes
Professionals	Diagnosis	Clinical
Facilities	Therapy	Functional
Technologies	Interaction	Perception
Organizations	Leadership	
Resources	Management	

Donabedian's work was the first to describe an approach to assessing quality through a systems framework. However, the model is very basic and does not sufficiently describe interrelationships. This led to the development of other models to illuminate the interrelationships necessary for quality performance.

A second framework used to understand TQM and quality improvement (TQM/QI) in complex systems is the Baldrige National Healthcare Criteria for Performance Excellence Framework depicted in **Figure 2-2**. The Baldrige Award was created in 1987, named for former U.S. Secretary of Commerce Malcolm Baldrige in tribute to his managerial ability. The award is given to organizations demonstrating a commitment to quality excellence. This model displays the principles of TQM/QI and shows the interrelationships among the structural, process, and outcome factors.

Figure 2-2. Baldrige Healthcare Criteria for Performance Excellence Framework

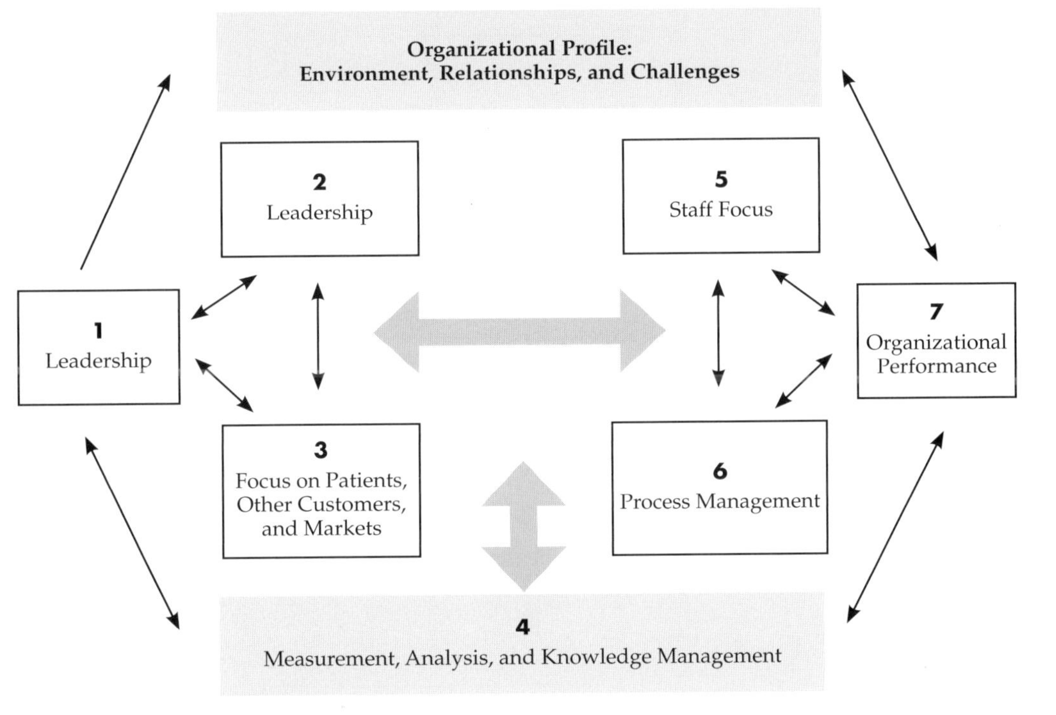

Source: Baldrige National Quality Program, 2005.

The organizational systems model depicted in **Figure 2-3** builds on these simpler models, further breaking down the elements and showing relationships among structure, process, and outcomes. The model begins at the top of the rectangle with formulation of mission, guiding principles, strategy, goals, and objectives; these give the organization direction and are the basis for strategy formulation. The "environment" box represents the multitude of stakeholders that must be satisfied and the arrow demonstrates that the environment can influence the direction the healthcare organization takes. Leadership is a critical process variable that influences the extent to which the structures (inputs) lead to desirable outcomes. The lower half of the diagram depicts subsystems of the organization or, in Donabedian's terms, *structural variables*. The lines connecting the various subsystems are meant

Figure 2-3. Organizational Systems Model

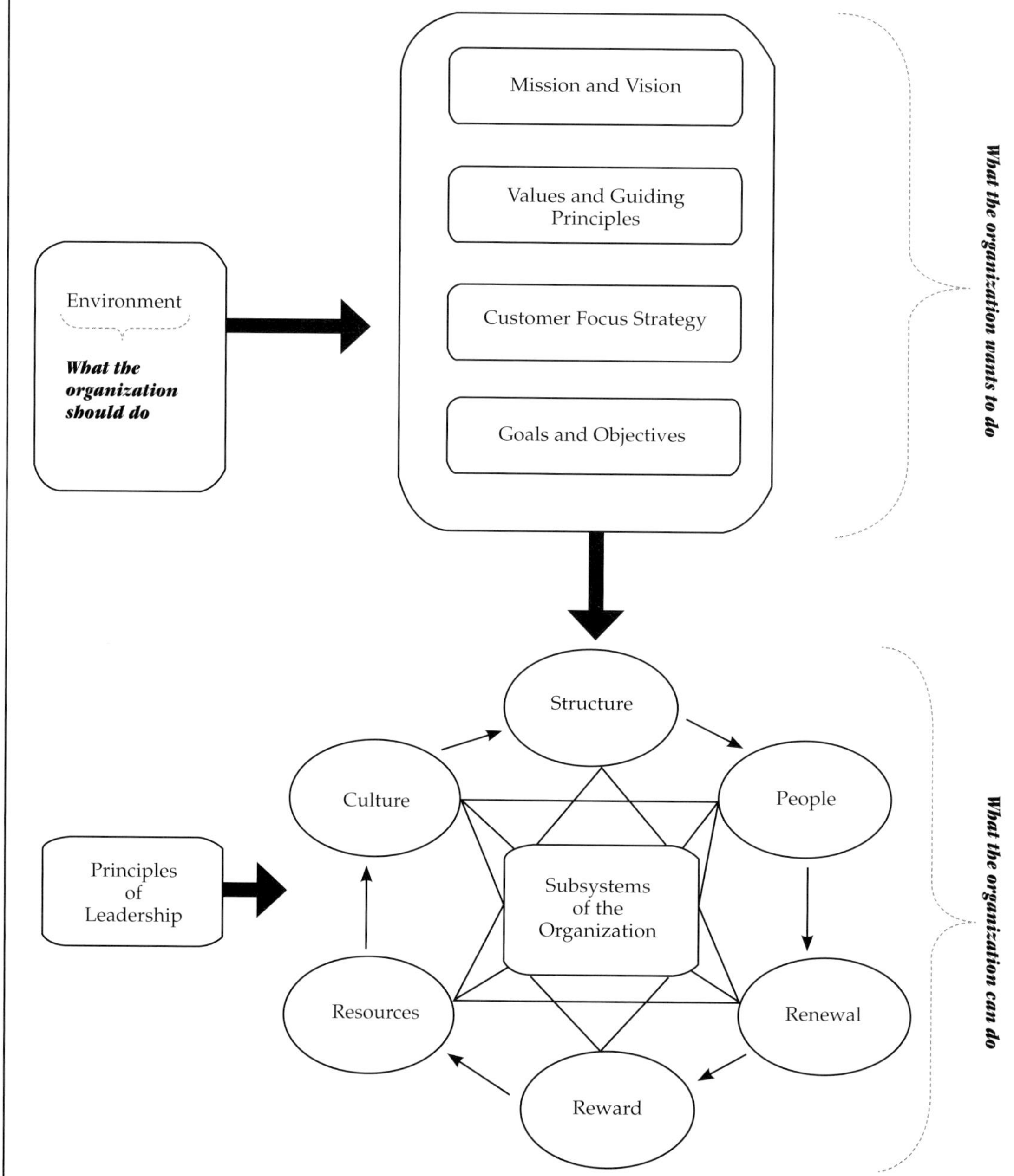

Sources: Axtell & Eckholdt, 1992; Kelly, 2003.

to demonstrate that subsystems are interdependent. Changes in one subsystem typically mean that changes must also occur in other subsystems to keep them aligned. This conceptualization of subsystems was suggested by Peters and Waterman (1982) more than 20 years ago but remains just as applicable today.

The IOM report *Crossing the Quality Chasm: A New Health System for the 21st Century* (CQHCA, 2001) provides a framework that identifies new rules for the healthcare system and contrasts these with the current approach (see **Table 2-2**). Thus, plans for the design or redesign of the organization should consider these new rules or guidelines.

Table 2-2. Rules for the 21st-Century Healthcare System

Current Approach	New Rule
• Care is based primarily on visits.	• Preference is given to professional roles over the system.
• Professional autonomy drives variability.	• Care is customized according to patient needs and values.
• Professionals control care.	• The patient is the source of control.
• Information is a record.	• Knowledge is shared and information flows freely.
• Decision making is based on training and experience.	• Decision making is evidence-based.
• "Do no harm" is an individual responsibility.	• Safety is a system priority.
• Confidentiality is necessary.	• Transparency is necessary.
• The system reacts to needs.	• Needs are anticipated.
• Cost reduction is sought.	• Waste is continuously decreased.
• Preference is given to professional roles over the system.	• Cooperation among clinicians is a priority.

Source: CQHCA, IOM, 2001, p. 67

III. Strategic Planning for Healthcare Quality: Guiding the Organization

"Without a strategy the organization is like a ship without a rudder, going around in circles." Joel Ross and Michael Kami (Thompson & Strickland, 1996)

The organizational systems design model serves as a roadmap for the remainder of the discussion on strategy and leadership. Each model component and the interrelationships are discussed in detail in the context of TQM/QI. The road to quality improvement begins with strategic planning.

A. Definition and Importance

The environment surrounding healthcare organizations is *dynamic* (changes frequently) and *complex* (with many constituents). External forces in healthcare have become increasingly more important since the mid-1990s with the focus on reform efforts and reduction in healthcare costs. The significant growth of managed care and its organizational entities (e.g., preferred provider organizations [PPOs], health maintenance organizations [HMOs], and preferred health organizations [PHOs]) accompanied by the significant shift away from the acute care hospital as a focus for delivery of care to subacute and ambulatory settings, has made strategic planning even more important.

Strategy is defined as "the plans and activities developed by an organization in pursuit of its goals and objectives, particularly in regard to positioning itself to meet external demands relative to its competition" (Shortell, Morrison, & Robbins, 1985, p. 220). Strategic planning is one way of coping with a dynamic and complex environment. The goals of strategic management (Ginter, et al., 2002) are to

- provide a framework for thinking about the "business"
- create a fit between the organization and its external environment
- provide a process for coping with change and organizational renewal
- foster anticipation, innovation, and excellence
- facilitate consistent decision making
- create organizational focus.

Quality has received a great deal of industry attention in recent years because organizations have come to realize that, to be successful, quality must be an integral part of the strategic plan.

B. Strategic Management Process

The strategic management process includes all the decisions and actions required to meet the strategic goals. **Figure 2-4** shows the steps in the strategic management process. Before a strategy is formulated, leaders consider what they want to do, what they should do, and what they can do (Luthans, Hodgetts, & Thompson, 1990). Consideration of these three issues leads to the development of a strategic plan.

1. What the Organization Wants To Do

a. Mission and Vision

Organizations must define what they want to accomplish in the future. *Mission* refers to the organization's purpose or reason for existing. It answers questions such as, "Why are we here?" "Whom do we serve?" and "What do we do?" For example, the mission of SSM Health Care, a Malcolm Baldrige National Quality Award recipient, is "Through our exceptional healthcare services, we reveal the healing presence of God." Its core values are compassion, respect, excellence, stewardship, and community (SSM Health Care, 2005). This provides a long-term direction for the organization.

Vision is an organization's statement of its goals for the future, described in measurable terms that clarify the direction for everyone in the organization. An organization's direction is built upon its mission and is guided by its vision.

b. Guiding Principles and Core Values

Guiding principles define the organization's attitudes and policies for employees and thereby help to direct the vision. Customer focus is a core value central to any improvement initiative. The *customer* is the person or entity that receives the process, product, or service and therefore defines the quality of products or services received. The key to performance improvement is knowing and understanding the customer. The following list displays other core values contained in the Baldrige National Quality Program Criteria for Performance and Excellence (Baldrige National Quality Program, 2004).

Figure 2-4. Strategic Management Process

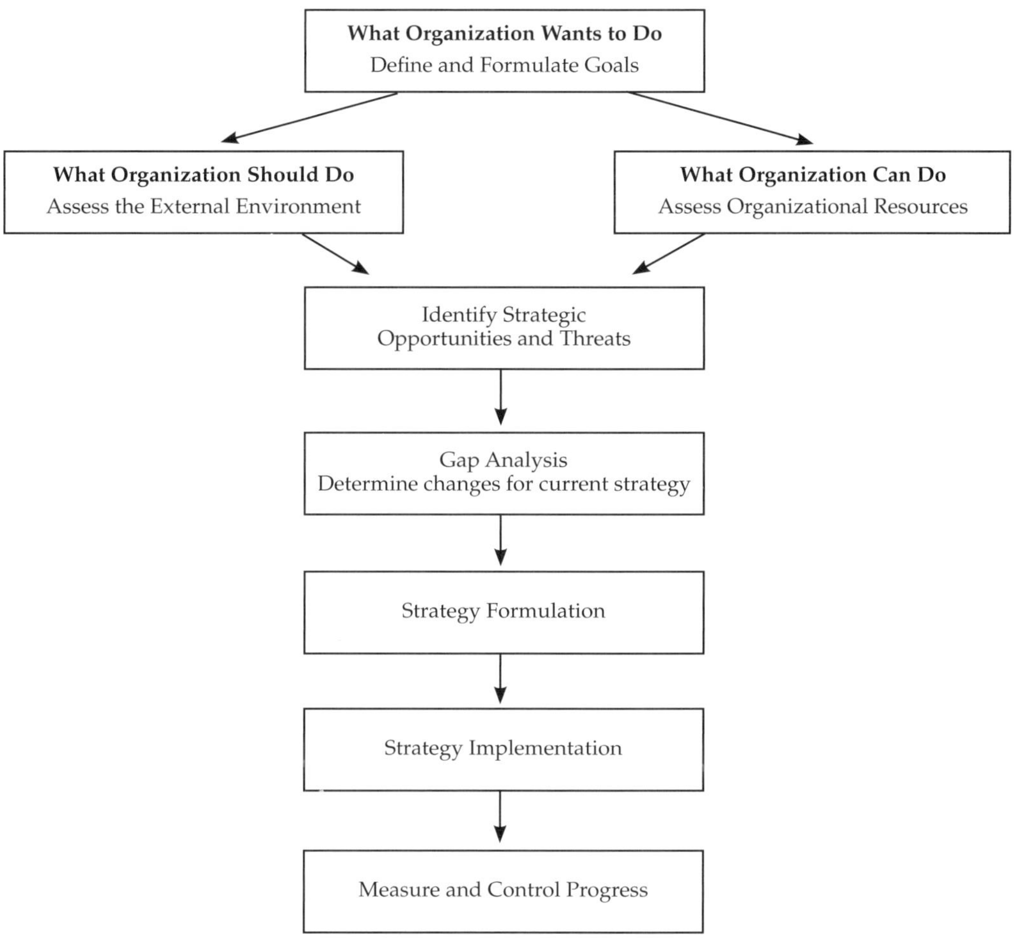

Adapted from Dunham & Pierce, 1989.

- visionary leadership
- customer-driven excellence
- organizational and personal learning
- valuing employees and partners
- agility
- focus on the future
- managing for innovation
- management by fact
- public responsibility and citizenship
- focus on results and creating value
- systems perspective.

c. Goals and Objectives

Goals and objectives are essential components of any planning process; they guide actions and serve as a yardstick for measuring the organization's progress and performance. Bill Hewlett, co-founder of Hewlett-Packard, once observed, "You cannot manage what you cannot measure...and what gets measured gets done" (House & Price, 1991, p. 93). There sometimes is confusion over the terms *goal* and *objective*; they differ with respect to scope and specificity. In general, goals are broad, general statements specifying a purpose or desired outcome and may be more abstract in nature than objectives (one goal can have several objectives).

Establishing goals is the initial step in the strategic planning process and sets the direction for the activities to follow. In general, goals need to be

- observable
- measurable
- challenging but attainable
- controllable
- visible
- time-limited.

Objectives are specific statements that detail how the goals will be achieved; they therefore are relatively narrow and concrete. Objectives represent the organization's commitment to achieving specific outcomes. They should be written as action-oriented statements, outlining specific activities to be carried out and measurable and observable qualitative or quantitative performance outcomes. Examples of a mission statement, strategic goals, and strategic objectives can be found in **Table 2-3**.

Table 2-3. Examples of Mission, Goals, and Objectives

Mission Statement	As a teaching hospital and critical member of the community, our mission is to provide high-quality, innovative healthcare services to all members of our community regardless of race, religion, nationality, or ability to pay. We are dedicated to educating clients with an emphasis on preventive healthcare.
Strategic Goals	To be recognized as one of the top healthcare providers in the community.
	Establish outreach program for management of chronic illness.
	Develop state-of-the-art program for breast cancer detection and treatment.
	Reduce project costs by 15%.
Strategic Objectives	Hire highly skilled nursing staff and set minimum nurse-to-patient ratios to reduce staff turnover.
	Obtain communication technology to allow distance education of clients and providers.
	Provide education and time reimbursement for physicians to train in innovative breast cancer technology.
	Control costs by using computerized planning tools (e.g., Program Evaluation Review Technique [PERT]).

The following are some general guidelines to use when writing objectives (Fisher & Samways, 1985):

- Keep the statements short and simple.
- State the end results or desired outcome and not just an activity.
- Specify the action to be taken, the condition under which the action is to be performed, and the criteria for successful completion.
- Write precisely in order to determine to what extent the objectives have been accomplished and what remains to be accomplished.
- Prioritize the objectives.

Once goals are developed at the executive level, there must be corresponding goals and objectives for other levels in the organization, for example, the business level and functional level (e.g., human resources, research and development); and the unit or departmental level (e.g., nursing, radiology, pharmacy). All levels should have both long-term and short-term goals and objectives.

2. Assessment of the External Environment (What the Organization Should Do)

Once the objectives have been established (or revised), the organization must look at the external environment. On the roadmap, the environment is shown to influence what the organization wants to do. This is because all organizations must adapt to the forces of the external environment in order to survive, stretch, and grow. In other words, the organization is one system among a variety of other systems in the external environment. Adaptation includes maintaining good relationships with key constituents who can influence its ability to meet the stated objectives. **Figure 2-5** depicts the various constituents whose needs must be met and balanced with the needs of other stakeholders. The outer ring pertains to the overall environment in which the organization exists. A variety of factors, including sociocultural, political and legal, economic, technological, global, and demographic forces indirectly influence the organization. For example, economic forces can influence the amount of resources available to organizations (e.g., labor,

Figure 2-5. Potential Environmental Influences on Quality Improvement

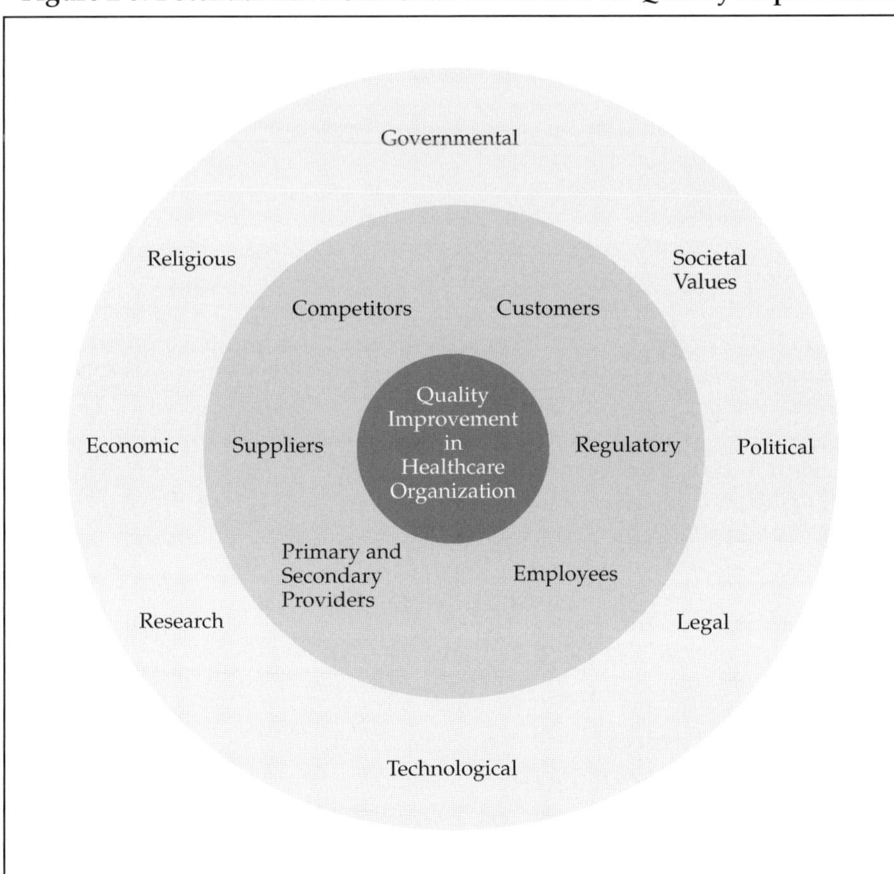

capital). This is why organizations must scan the general external environment looking for threats to, or opportunities for, meeting strategic goals and objectives.

The second ring represents the immediate environment in which the organization operates. With respect to TQM/QI, the key constituent is the customer! However, other constituents also are important. For example, the entity through which the patient acquires healthcare insurance (typically an employer), payers, and regulatory agencies also are key stakeholders.

3. Assessment of the Internal Environment (What the Organization Can Do)

Once the organization has established what it wants to do and what it should do based on assessment of the external environment, it needs to know what it can do. This requires an examination of the internal environment that looks at the resources, capabilities, and core competencies of the organization. Resources can be tangible (human, financial, physical) or intangible (reputation). For example, if an organization wants to be a leader in breast cancer detection and treatment, it must have qualified staff and equipment. (Resources are addressed in more detail later in this module.)

4. Strategy Formulation

Based on the strategic goals, objectives, and evaluation of external and internal environments, strategic opportunities and threats are identified. Generally, organizations perform a gap analysis in which they evaluate the extent to which the present strategy would have to be changed in order to meet the goals and objectives. Strategy formulation clearly stipulates actions to be taken to achieve goals. In the systems model (Figure 2-3), this is indicated by the arrows pointing to the lower half of the rectangle, describing the various subsystems in the organization that will undertake these actions to help the organization reach its goals.

5. Strategy Implementation

The various units and departments develop their own strategies that will contribute to the overall goals and objectives of the organization. There are a number of approaches that top management can take to integrate TQM/QI with strategic planning and to ensure that plans and strategies are being carried out. *Hoshin planning* (a Japanese term that means policy deployment) is one approach for integration.

Hoshin planning is a component of the TQM/QI system used to ensure that the vision set forth by top management is being translated into planning objectives and actions that both management and employees will take to accomplish long-term organizational strategic goals (see **Figure 2-6**). "The primary reason to undertake Hoshin planning is to focus effort and resources on those few strategies and processes that will best achieve the organization's survival and vision, and to develop an effective process to align the goals and efforts of the organization" (Gaucher & Coffey, 1993, p. 492). The planning typically is performed at three levels: general (senior management), intermediate (middle management), and detailed (implementation teams).

6. Measure and Control

In this last step of strategic planning, management seeks to evaluate the extent to which the strategy is accomplishing the goals set forth in the first step of strategic planning and takes any necessary corrective action. Actual performance is evaluated and compared to the performance goals and objectives established as part of the strategic plan. Gaps between desired performance and actual performance require

Figure 2-6. Core Hoshin Planning Process

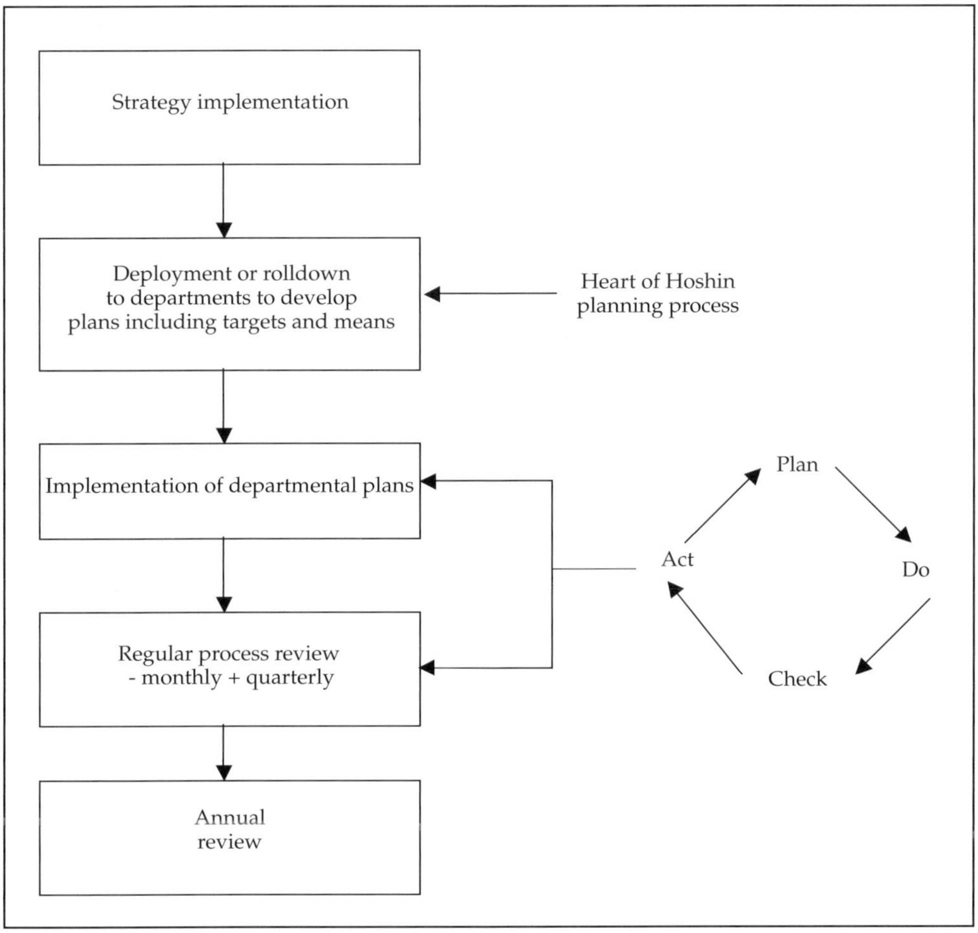

action. Many factors influence the effectiveness of strategy. Among the most important is the need for effective leadership.

IV. Leadership: Translating Strategic Goals into Quality Outcomes

A. The Board's Role in TQM/QI

The organization's board of trustees bears ultimate responsibility for setting policy, for financial and strategic direction, and for the quality of care provided by all of its practitioners. Together with the organization's management and medical staff leaders, the board sets priorities for TQM/QI activities.

The development of meaningful board involvement in TQM/QI requires assessment of the board's knowledge regarding TQM/QI. This is a key role of healthcare quality professionals, who are responsible for organizing and coordinating quality management and performance improvement activities for the organization and its medical staff. Healthcare quality professionals can promote the board's commitment to quality by providing useful information in a format easily understood by members who may lack familiarity with healthcare terminology and procedures.

The American Hospital Association outlined six broad categories of responsibilities and functions for the board and top leaders (Orlikoff, 1990):

- *Organization*—The governing body or board is responsible for organizing itself effectively, for selecting a qualified chief executive officer (CEO), and for ensuring that the medical staff is appropriately organized.
- *Public policy and external relationships*—The governing body is responsible for maintaining productive external relationships and for influencing public policies related to healthcare.
- *Strategic planning*—The governing body is responsible for and has the authority to develop a strategic plan and determine the organization's mission, goals, and objectives.
- *Resource management*—The governing body has oversight for the organization's resources, including development, utilization, and maintenance.
- *Human resource development*—The governing body is responsible for the protection and enhancement of the institution's human resources.
- *Education and research*—The governing body is responsible for ensuring access to education and research programs that support the organization's mission. The development of meaningful board involvement is a process that requires careful planning, thoughtful implementation, and continual refinement. This process consists of assessing current knowledge, developing a plan based on that assessment, and conducting ongoing evaluation of the board's effectiveness.

For practical purposes, day-to-day leadership is delegated to the CEO and senior management, elected or appointed members of the medical staff (e.g., chairs), and administrative and clinical staff (e.g., healthcare quality professionals).

B. Fundamental Principles of Leadership

Leadership is the ability to influence an individual or group toward achievement of goals (Robbins, 2001). Leadership and management are not identical. Leadership is determining the correct direction or path, whereas *management* is doing the correct things to stay on that path. Kotter (1990) notes that management is about coping with complexity through planning and budgeting; setting of goals; organizing, staffing, and creating a structure to foster goal attainment; setting up mechanisms for monitoring; and controlling results. In contrast, leaders are responsible for coping with change by developing a vision for change and aligning the subsystems of the organization. Both strong leadership and management are necessary for high performance. Some individuals are great leaders but poor managers and vice versa; in some cases, an individual may be successful in both roles.

C. Leadership Framework

There are many frameworks for leadership. As is true with the systems framework, it often is less important which particular framework is selected than simply to have one to guide behavior. Deming believed that managers were responsible for optimizing the system. According to the systems model in Figure 2-3, "optimizing" would involve aligning the subsystems of the organization. What types of leadership practices are essential to this process?

Practices of exemplary leaders were explored by Kouzes and Posner (2002) who identified five important general practices: (1) inspire a shared vision, (2) challenge the process, (3) enable others to act, (4) model the way, and (5) encourage the heart.

These principles are generic and, thus, applicable to any type of organization. A brief overview of these practices is presented below.

Inspire a shared vision. For any change to be successful, leaders must provide a vision for TQM/QI and influence people to share that vision. This means getting people to accept the core values underlying TQM/QI by developing a strong culture for quality improvement (discussed further in the "Culture" subsystem).

Challenge the system. Challenging the system means acting as a change agent for that vision. It also means recognizing good ideas and demonstrating a willingness to stretch and grow in order to improve the quality of care. This, too, involves adoption of core values as a learning organization.

Enable others to act. The third leadership practice is enabling others to act by sharing decision making and power. Along with sharing power, "enabling" involves having an appropriate structural design and resources to support TQM/QI initiatives (discussed further in the "Structure" subsystem).

Model the way. Much behavior is learned through role modeling. Leaders who expect employees to make changes to support quality improvement must model those desired behaviors; actions speak louder than words.

Encourage the heart. The last practice is critical. Change is difficult, even if it is done for the "right" reasons. "Encouraging the heart" means recognizing contributions employees make and celebrating the core values and victories. The most important point of any reward system is to reward the desired behaviors (discussed further in "Rewards" subsystems).

Leaders use these five practices to keep subsystems aligned. However, leaders must first get people to support a vision of quality. One way this occurs is to develop a strong culture of quality improvement.

V. Aligning Culture To Support Quality

A. Definition and Importance of Culture

Culture has been defined as the social "glue" that holds people together (Siehl & Martin, 1981). At the heart of culture is the notion of shared values (what is important) and behavioral "norms" (the way things are done; Rokeach, 1973). Cultures are described as strong when the core values are intensely held and widely shared. Strong culture

- provides a sense of identity for employees; commitment to something larger than themselves
- enhances cooperation
- creates a system of informal rules spelling out how people are expected to behave
- creates distinctions between organizations, allowing for a definite competitive advantage to develop.

B. Elements of Culture

Culture has both hidden and visible elements. Hidden elements are values and norms; whereas visible elements include symbols; language, slogans, and brands; ritual and ceremonies; stories, legends, and myths; and heroes.

Values and norms. The core values reflected in the Baldrige National Quality Program were previously discussed. The role of leaders is to inspire commitment to these underlying quality values.

Symbols. Symbols are things that represent an idea. The purpose of symbols is to reflect the culture, trigger values and norms, and help people make sense of their organization. For example, one hospital wanted to strengthen the value for reporting adverse events. To do this, staff wore buttons that said: "We care, We report, We learn."

Language, slogans, and brands. Language and slogans are intended to convey cultural meaning to employees and/or stakeholders. They should be easy to learn, remember, and repeat (e.g., "Quality is Job 1"). Brands help build loyalty to a product or service.

Rituals and ceremonies. Rituals and ceremonies reinforce an organization's core values and goals, thereby strengthening culture.

Stories, legends, and myths. Stories, legends, and myths are narrative examples repeated among employees to inform (often new) employees about culture. Stories are based on fact; legends are based on facts but embellished; myths are consistent with the culture but are not based on fact.

Heroes. Heroes are company role models whose ideals, character, and support of the organizational culture highlight the values and norms a company wishes to reinforce. Heroes provide a role model for success. By design or default, an organization develops a culture. It is better to actively direct the evolution of that culture than to try and change a strong culture that is not aligned with the goals of quality improvement.

C. Assessing Culture

How can it be determined whether TQM/QI is a core value in an organization? Experts in the field of culture suggest posing the following questions (Schein, 1992; Schneider, 1990):

- Does the leader pay attention to, measure, and control quality on a regular basis?
- Are scarce resources allocated to TQM/QI?
- Are behaviors supporting QI rewarded?
- Do staff knowledge, skills, and behaviors important for QI figure into decisions regarding recruitment, selection, and promotion?
- Is active involvement in TQM/QI activities one measure of status in the organization?
- Are people spending time on TQM/QI?
- Does staff frequently discuss TQM/QI?
- Is the prevailing attitude toward TQM/QI positive or negative?

D. Strengthening Culture for Quality Improvement

Many actions for strengthening a quality culture flow from the above questions. First, leaders must show visible support through such actions as

- making QI everyone's responsibility
- having an annual budget for TQM/QI
- making QI part of the strategic planning process
- rewarding behaviors that support TQM/QI.

Second, the visible elements of culture must receive attention. For example, the following must be accomplished.

- Old, negative stories about QI that are acting as barriers to cultural change must be replaced with new, positive ones.
- Symbols to reinforce values critical to quality need to be created. Rituals that reinforce values critical to quality need to be established.
- Leaders must celebrate successes relating to QI.

Finally, leaders must be persistent! Culture takes a long time to change.

Although inspiring people to a vision is critical, leaders must also enable others to achieve goals and objectives. One way to enable others is to structure or design the organization in a way that supports quality improvement.

VI. Aligning Structure To Support Quality

A. Definition and Importance

Designing an organization is similar to designing a house. "Like the physical structure of a house, organizational structure identifies and distinguishes the individual parts of an organization and ties these pieces together to define an integrated whole. Organizational structure differs from the physical structure of a house, however, in that it encompasses more than inanimate characteristics of walls, doors, and windows. Organizational structure includes the interaction patterns that link people to people and people to work, and unlike a house, structural dimensions of organizations frequently change and evolve" (Dunham & Pierce, 1989, p. 399).

B. Basic Structural Elements

Evans and Dean (2003) state that six basic structural elements have great influence on quality:

- focus on processes
- recognition of internal customers
- reduction of hierarchy
- creation of a team-based organization
- use of steering committees
- development of an agile organization.

1. Focus on Processes

A focus on processes concerns the structural elements referred to as *departmentation*; that is, how jobs are grouped together. Jobs can be grouped by function, product or service, geography, and process or customer. TQM/QI tends toward process structure as opposed to functional, supporting both Deming and Juran, who note that quality issues more often arise from processes than from worker issues. This also is true of patient safety, where it has been demonstrated that most errors occur as a function of faulty systems as opposed to incompetent staff.

Core processes are those that are critical to customer satisfaction. Particularly important to quality of care are the processes relating to risk management (RM), utilization management (UM), and case management.

a. Risk Management

Definition and importance. "Risk management for healthcare entities can be defined as an organized effort to identify, assess, and reduce, where appropriate, risk to patients, visitors, staff and organizational assets (Kavaler & Spiegel, 1997, p. 3). The goal of RM in any organization is to protect the organization from financial losses, which may arise because of the risks to which it is exposed.

History and evolution of risk management. In the 1970s, RM was the initial reaction to continually increasing litigation. However, as litigation continued to rise, RM assumed a more proactive role in attempting to reduce the incidents of unsafe care. **Table 2-4** outlines the evolution of RM.

Table 2-4. Evolution of Healthcare Risk Management

Then	Now
Number one goal: to protect financial resources and reputation.	Number one goal: improve patient safety; minimize risk of harm to patient through better understanding of systemic factors that inhibit caregiver's ability to provide safe care.
Paper occurrence form required.	Variety of methods to report: paper form, electronic form, telephone call, anonymous reporting, person-to-person reporting.
Investigate only the serious occurrences.	Encourage reporting of "near misses" and investigate and discuss the potential.
Interview staff one on one when there is an adverse incident.	Have root cause analysis meetings with the entire team of caregivers.
Information from investigation kept confidential.	Develop corrective action, share with patient safety committee and others within the organization.
Blame and train.	Perform a criticality analysis chart and determine the root cause of the "near miss" or the adverse occurrence.
Talk to the patient/patient's family only if necessary and be vague about findings.	Advise physician to speak directly with the patient/family and talk with them about any unexpected outcomes and errors; keep them apprised of steps taken to make environment safe for next patient.
Work with department involved to develop corrective action.	Work with team to develop a patient safety improvement plan.
Assume that action is taken to correct the problem that occurred, notice only when it happens again that no action was taken.	Monitor the patient safety improvement plan to determine that changes have been initiated and that the changes have made a difference.
Keep patients in the dark about risk management and occurrence reporting.	Establish ongoing patient safety education; publish patient safety bulletins that address specific patient safety issues and the organization's approach to managing them; provide opportunity for patients to identify methods of improving patient safety and to share them with administration.

Source: Kuhn & Youngberg, Quality and safety in health care, *2002. Reprinted with permission.*

Clinical risk management. A healthcare risk manager must consider such things as regulatory compliance; safety management; credentialing; client-provider relations; publicity and media coverage; and, most importantly, patient care. In this way, RM and TQM/QI are closely related. Both are keenly interested in maintaining or exceeding the applicable standard of care. Thus, in a healthcare organization, the term *clinical risk management* sometimes is used to indicate the concern and interest taken in clinical care provided to patients, clients, and other customers.

Basic risk management functions. The risk manager is an important asset to the organization, as that individual is charged with risk identification, risk evaluation, and application of techniques to reduce risks. Duties vary widely by organization, but the basic RM functions are

- maintenance and monitoring of effective incident reporting and occurrence screening programs
- claims management
- clinical and administrative responsibilities such as policy review, credentialing, contract review, internal and external reporting, and education

- collaboration with the organization's safety officer (the risk manager may be the safety officer in smaller organizations)
- collaboration with financial office staff regarding insurance and other methods of risk financing
- regulatory compliance.

Process of risk management. The process of RM includes five basic steps:

- Step 1: Identify exposure to accidental loss.
- Step 2: Examine various RM techniques to reduce exposure.
- Step 3: Select the best RM technique for the situation.
- Step 4: Implement the chosen technique.
- Step 5: Monitor the effectiveness of the chosen technique.

Risk management plan. A healthcare organization typically has a plan explaining its RM philosophy. Often the RM plan is integrated with the quality management plan because the two processes are interdependent. Important plan elements include

- purpose and board statement of support of RM
- scope of the program, authority, and confidentiality assertions
- data collection and reporting mechanisms (both internal and external)
- integration with quality management and program effectiveness reviews.

Education and skills for risk managers. It is helpful for risk managers to have some clinical knowledge, because she or he must review care and provide guidance to clinical providers of care. As risk managers must review defense counsel work and legal documents, they should have some knowledge of healthcare law and have a thorough understanding of the legal system. Finally, understanding the insurance industry is important because risk managers help make decisions regarding various insurance coverages such as hospital professional liability, general liability, and workers' compensation.

b. Utilization Management

Definition, goals, and objectives. Pressure to manage resources has increased in recent years owing to the high costs of healthcare. UM is an organized, comprehensive approach to analyze, direct, and conserve organizational resources, so as to provide care that is high in quality, efficient, and cost-effective.

History/evolution. The need to develop a UM program in the United States emerged in response to the changing needs and expectations of consumers. With the return of veterans following World War II (WWII) came the need for more medical services. In addition to more services, the population required a greater distribution of those services.

Prior to WWII, insurance coverage was inconsistent, scarce, and provided shallow coverage at best. With these new services, health insurance began to take form. As the public began to perceive access to healthcare as a right, not a privilege, two transformations occurred: responsibility for payment was removed from the consumer, and responsibility for controlling costs was removed from providers (hospitals, clinics, and physicians).

The need for some type of national health plan was identified and led to the establishment in 1966 of two federal programs: Medicare and Medicaid. As senior citizens retired, a need to provide their insurance coverage was identified and led to the Social Security Act of 1965. This provided medical coverage to those over 65 without private insurance. Once again, reimbursement for care was based on charges; therefore, no motivation existed for either provider or consumer to control or direct resource consumption.

By the 1970s, there was a proliferation of medical technology. To avoid charges of underserving their communities, every hospital had to have the latest equipment. The government could not continue to meet the spiraling costs of healthcare and determined to initiate some controls. The rationale included the following beliefs: healthcare consumers could not adequately judge service quality or necessity, there was a duty to protect the public from fraud and abuse, and consumers and providers were insensitive to costs.

The government's response was an attempt to regulate the healthcare industry with the following measures:

- development of the professional standard review organizations (now known as quality improvement organizations [QIOs])
- Certificate of Need (CON) program
- health systems agencies (HSAs)
- Medicare physician charge index.

The CON programs at the federal level were discontinued in 1986. Many states, however, continue to fund CON programs, which are time-consuming, costly, and, to some extent, quite political. CON programs and other regulatory strategies did little to solve the problems of control and direction of resource consumption, and costs continued to rise dramatically.

In 1983 with the passage of the Social Security amendments introducing the Tax Equity and Fiscal Responsibility Act of 1982 (TEFRA) legislation, a major change was directed at healthcare reimbursement. TEFRA legislation created the following

- a prospective pricing system that was based on diagnosis-related groups (DRGs), for Medicare hospital patients
- a defined cost-per-discharge methodology with reimbursement limits
- incentives to increase the number of discharges, to decrease length of stay (LOS) and ancillary service usage, to shift care to alternate settings, and to permit the development of alternative delivery systems such as HMOs and PPOs
- Medicare risk contracting by federally qualified HMOs.

In December 2003, President Bush signed into law the Medicare Prescription Drug, Improvement and Modernization Act of 2003. The purpose of this legislation is to improve healthcare to senior citizens by offering a prescription drug benefit to help with medication costs. In addition, this act allows seniors more choices in selecting a health plan, including better coverage for preventive care.

Public demand for more efficient use of resources while providing access to all in need of services has created a movement for healthcare reform. Comprehensive UM programs will continue to be important and will have an impact on the viability of every organization.

Program concepts/process. The overall function of a UM program is to facilitate the delivery of high-quality, low-cost, efficient, and effective care to all patients, regardless of the treatment setting. UM is responsible for a wide variety of tasks, including the following:

- *Medical necessity appropriateness review.* This element is an integral component of the UM department's daily function. Using targets established by the organization and medical necessity criteria (e.g., Interqual's Severity of Illness/Intensity of Service) developed and/or approved by the medical staff and the governing body; each patient's encounter is reviewed against the criteria.

- *Discharge planning and monitoring.* To move the patient through the healthcare system appropriately, and to provide the patient with the appropriate level of service delivery at each point in the continuum of care, timely and effective discharge planning is paramount. The UM program should include monitoring and facilitation of this process.
- *Overutilization and underutilization surveillance.* Identification of over- and underutilization is fundamental to every UM program and requires professionals to review cases for appropriate use of resources and evaluate the impact on quality outcomes.
- *Quality of care and liability problems.* During the course of review, quality of care and risk/liability issues should be identified and reported promptly for timely follow-up.
- *Financial issues.* Utilization programs obtain concurrent financial as well as clinical data on all applicable cases to be useful. This "data marriage" not only educates providers about the cost of treating their patients, but also provides the leadership and the governing body with case mix and cost data information in addition to statistics on LOS, complications, and mortality.
- *Medical/organization staff education.* There are many opportunities to provide education on resource management, including regular in-service programs, participation and reporting at department/unit meetings, newsletters, the organization's Intranet, and one-on-one communication.
- *Leadership/governing body reporting.* A successful UM program includes a plan consistent with the organization's strategic plan. Reports of UM indicators frequently are incorporated in the quarterly quality reports ("dashboards") to the board. Healthcare quality professionals can be instrumental in suggesting which parameters to present and which data display formats to use.

Program design. There are no rigid guidelines with respect to the structure of the UM function; however, most traditional methods involve a formal committee that typically includes a physician and organizational representatives (e.g., finance, nursing, administration, social services, discharge planning, and high-volume ancillary) who review the issues and forward recommendations.

Physician advisers. The role of the physician adviser is pivotal to any UM program, providing critical peer review and serving as a liaison for the medical staff and UM. Typically, a physician adviser will be consulted when the efforts of the UM/case management coordinator have failed to resolve an issue. Organizations should have a written position description for the physician adviser that details the responsibility and accountability described above.

c. Case Management

History. As the delivery of care becomes more complex, care tends to be more disjointed. Case management is one method to coordinate diverse elements involved in the delivery of healthcare to the individual. Case management is not a new concept; its roots in the United States can be traced to 1863, when the Commonwealth of Massachusetts established the first Board of Charities to coordinate public human service and conserve public funds used to care for the poor and sick. Case management increased in importance after WWII (and again after the creation of the President's Commission on Mental Retardation in 1962) as a way to extend and improve services. In the 1970s, the Service Interaction Targets for Opportunities Program utilized case management to integrate social and health services for patients, thereby formalizing case management as a reimbursable, distinct service. With the passage of the Omnibus Budget Reconciliation Act of 1981, prospective, DRG-based payment for medical care of the aged made case management attractive to hospitals.

Case management models. Many models are available for case management. The American Nurses Association describes 12 different models that can be grouped into four basic categories:

- reimbursement-based models, which focus on controlling healthcare costs through integration and coordination of services
- institution-based models, which typically are found in hospitals, home healthcare agencies, and nursing homes; the goal is to tie together the related services within and outside the organization to provide patients with optimal care
- social services, based as part of the social welfare service
- private management-based models, which usually are employed by patients or families to plan financial and healthcare needs.

Importance of case management. Coordination of a patient's care—from preventive interventions, to more intensive modalities during an episode of illness, through the recovery phase—promotes a continuum of care that is critical to patient satisfaction and efficient use of resources. It is the role of the case manager to ensure that only medically appropriate and cost-conscious care is provided to patients. The case manager maintains an overview of the case and helps the primary care provider maintain an objective ongoing assessment of the patient's healthcare needs. The case manager also is responsible for ensuring continuity of care from hospital to home, home to hospital, or hospital to subacute or long-term care facility. Case management has been demonstrated to increase nursing and medical efficiency and increase quality of patient care.

The case management process. The case management process consists of intake and assessment, development of a care plan, case coordination, discharge planning, and quality management.

- Intake and assessment begins with admission to a particular service. In addition to observing the patient, reviewing the medical history, and conducting a physical examination, the healthcare provider also observes and assesses socioeconomic, cultural, cognitive, and emotional factors that may affect the patient.
- A comprehensive care plan is developed after the initial assessment using input from all members of the care team. The plan of care should contain
  - a treatment plan established by the healthcare practitioner in cooperation with the primary care provider, the patient, and family
  - clearly defined, measurable short- and long-term goals and expected outcomes with time frames for completion
  - a plan and tools for patient and family education
  - case coordination and referral information.
- Discharge planning begins at the time of admission, with input from all stakeholders (e.g., patient, family, physician, primary care nurse). A discharge plan should include information relating to
  - care coordination among the various case managers (e.g., hospital, subacute or long-term care, home healthcare, and private insurance)
  - involvement of ancillary services (e.g., physical therapy) after discharge and home healthcare/therapy plan or follow-up counseling
  - expected discharge date
  - goals to be met before discharge

  - specific instructions (e.g., equipment use, preventive measures)
  - specifics regarding follow-up plans with the primary care provider.
- The case manager ensures effectiveness of care through monitoring outcomes and working closely with other healthcare professionals to develop effectiveness indicators.

For these important programs to succeed, potential barriers must be addressed, including the following: lack of communication or understanding about the existence or purpose of the program; lack of recognized authority or support by administration and/or medical staff; and unwillingness of organization, physicians, or staff to change practices. Module Four addresses change and resistance to change.

2. Recognition of Internal Customers

A second important structural element in TQM/QI is recognizing internal customers. Every process has both internal and external customers. Most people readily understand the concept of being a supplier of goods to an external customer. However, the idea of internal customers is equally important to TQM/QI.

An employee can be a customer when she or he receives material, information, or services from others in the organization. Conversely, an employee also can be a supplier, when she or he provides material, information, or services to others in the organization or to external customers. For example, when a nurse sends a specimen to the laboratory, the nurse is the supplier and the laboratory is the customer. When the laboratory sends a report back to the nurse, the laboratory is the supplier and the nurse is the customer. Just as there are suppliers to internal customers, those internal customers can, in turn, be suppliers to external customers. This approach can help to

- remind those departments that do not have direct contact with external customers that they are still a critical link to customer satisfaction
- improve relationships
- make the work process flow smoothly
- avert potential bottlenecks.

Table 2-5 provides an example of an approach one organization followed to ensure the recognition of internal customers. Notice that the customer service standard pledge reflects the values necessary to make quality improvement a reality (e.g., teamwork, information-sharing).

3. Reduction in Hierarchy

One direct approach leaders can take to enable others to act is to modify the structure of the organization by reducing the hierarchy. Hierarchy relates to the number of managerial levels in the organization. There has been a trend in recent years toward a significant "flattening" (reduction in the number of levels), with more focus on employee participation through cross-functional collaboration (usually in the form of teams). Flatter organizations also include the abolishment of silos—replacing department-specific focus with interdepartmental and cross-functional work.

Flatter organizations typically require decentralized decision making whereby the authority and responsibility for making decisions are spread throughout the organization. But how is power shared in an equitable way? In recent years the topic of shared governance—the mechanism for equitably integrating the interests of a variety of groups in the organization—has received a great deal of attention. Shared governance has been linked to employee satisfaction and is necessary in healthcare systems due to the following factors:

Table 2-5. Customer Service Standards and Pledge

Internal Customers: Our Pledge To Each Other (fellow employees and hospital personnel)			
Respect me and my job	**We are all professionals**	**Work/communicate with me**	**Smile—it's contagious**
Our need: Respect *Our response:* I understand the need and I will • acknowledge you • be sensitive to your point of view • thank you for a job well done • value your time and priorities • discuss my concerns with you in private • value your job and its contribution to the organization • treat you as I would like to be treated • speak to you in a pleasant tone in person or on the phone	*Our need:* Professionalism *Our response:* I understand the need to represent the hospital in a professional manner and I will • take responsibility for my actions • protect confidential information about patients and fellow employees • look professional in dress, grooming, and manner • coach others when necessary • follow through on my promise to you	*Our need:* I understand the need for teamwork and I will • pitch in and offer to help you whenever possible • ask for your input before making a decision that may affect you • talk to you directly instead of talking to others secretly if I have a concern • listen to you, offer positive advice, and not interrupt until you are finished • recognize that everyone has a valid opinion • seek out information and share what I have learned	*Our need:* Positive attitude *Our response:* I understand the need for a positive work environment, and I will • be sensitive to the effects my actions have on others • replace criticism with positive ideas • try to see things through the other person's eyes • attempt to leave any personal problems at home • coach my coworkers in portraying a positive attitude • project a caring and concerned attitude

Source: Baird, Customer service in health care, *2000. Copyright ©2000 Jossey-Bass Publishers. Reprinted with permission of John Wiley & Sons, Inc.*

- Increased complexity regarding point of care—old hierarchical structures don't work.
- Information and knowledge explosion—patients have a multitude of independent care providers; no one has complete control. There must be mechanisms to allow people to act together.
- No healthcare organization can "own, control or unilaterally mandate all of the service linkages and connections necessary to serve a specific population" (Porter-O'Grady, Hawkins, & Parker, 1997, p. 39).

Principles of governance include issues relating to partnership, equity, accountability, and ownership (Porter-O'Grady, Hawkins, & Parker, 1997). In short, governance goes beyond providing infrastructure to support QI, such as membership on committees. To be successful, people must have power to make decisions and the prerequisite skills, such as those involved in conflict and negotiation, to participate.

Leaders, through their own management style, also can influence the degree to which employees share information, knowledge, rewards, and power in the organization. In general, there are three major participative styles:

- *Autocratic*—Leader is directive and controlling; employees have little discretionary power in their work.
- *Participative*—Leader allows employees some degree of autonomy in completing their work, seeks input from employees.
- *Empowering*—Leader shares power and decision making with employees, who have control over their work.

Deming (1986) maintains that improvements in quality are more likely to be realized when workers are empowered to solve problems, including changing processes and systems (most likely developed by management).

To work effectively, teams must be empowered. Empowerment enables people to

- take ownership of their jobs
- make decisions concerning their department or area
- take responsibility for their decisions
- add value to their jobs.

Empowerment does not mean that people can

- be free to do whatever they want
- reassign work that they do not want to do themselves
- disregard existing policies and practices
- avoid accountability for results
- fix, rescue, and give advice.

4. Creating a Team-Based Organization

Another important structural element for TQM/QI and process improvement is creating a team-based organization. Because patient care involves multiple disciplines, the linchpin for improvement is employees who have regular communication and contact that allows them to coordinate and problem solve to continuously improve quality of care. The organization must develop an infrastructure within which the cycle of improvement can operate. One feature of this infrastructure is teams.

a. What Is a Team?

A team is "a group of people who are interdependent with respect to information, resources, and skills and who seek to combine their efforts to achieve a common goal" (Thompson, 2000, p. 2).

b. Types of QI Teams

There are many types of teams. **Figure 2-7** provides a mechanism for classifying teams along five major dimensions: purpose or mission, time, degree of autonomy, authority structure, and physical presence (Greenberg & Baron, 2003). In TQM/QI, two teams are of great importance: steering committees (also referred to as *quality councils*) and QI teams.

Steering committees. Steering committees are permanent improvement teams consisting of cross-functional members. These committees are self-managed teams that provide direction and focus by identifying and prioritizing improvement opportunities in the organization. The role of the quality council is to sustain, facilitate, and expand the QI initiative based on the strategic plan. Membership should comprise top leaders in the organization, including medical staff. The main responsibilities of the quality council include

- lending legitimacy to the TQM/QI efforts
- maintaining organization focus on the identified goals
- fostering teamwork
- providing necessary resources (e.g., human, financial)
- formulating QI policies regarding quality priorities, participation, annual self-assessments, and reward and recognition systems.

Quality improvement teams. QI teams can be natural work teams—teams with members that work "permanently" as a team each day in order to complete the task. These teams can be cross-functional, as with an operating room team, or intact, such as a team of nurses in a particular unit. Autonomy varies, but there

Figure 2-7. Classification of Teams

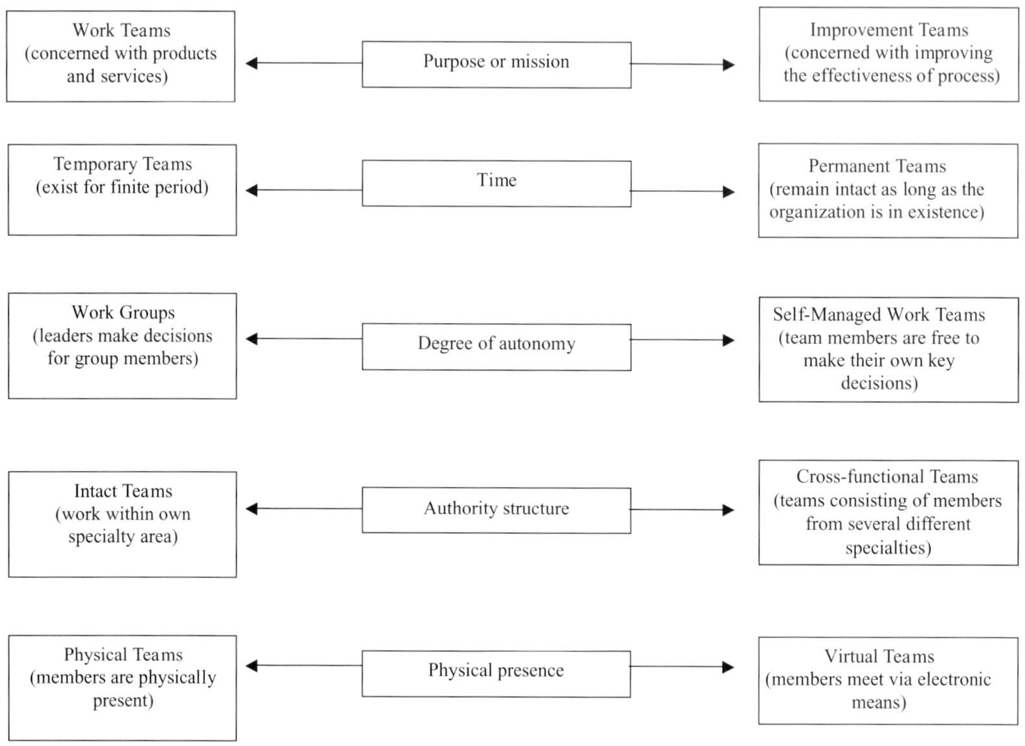

Source: Greenberg & Baron, Organizational behavior, *2003. Upper Saddle River, NJ: Prentice Hall. Reprinted with permission.*

typically is a leader. These teams can be temporary (e.g., brought together to solve a single problem) or permanent (e.g., continuous improvement teams).

c. When Should Teams Be Used?

Managers need to examine three aspects of the required task before deciding whether to use a team: task complexity, task interdependence, and task objectives (Luecke, 2004).

Tasks are considered to be complex when they involve large amounts of information, are performed under conditions of high uncertainty, contain many subtasks that require individuals with specialized skills and knowledge, and when there are no standardized procedures for completing the tasks. Teams are important as they bring larger numbers of specialized individuals to carry the burden and offer greater diverse inputs that are more likely to result in more alternatives generated and more creative solutions. Creativity is particularly important when there are no standardized procedures and the environment is uncertain.

Task interdependence means that the work of one person or persons is highly dependent upon the work of others. Patient care typically involves a multitude of disciplines that must coordinate their work and this requires intense communication. Teams therefore are appropriate, as this type of structure can foster communication among the various disciplines.

Finally, teams are appropriate to use when the task objectives are clear and time-bound. One approach for making task objectives clear is to develop a team charter. The charter should contain information regarding (Schwarz, Landis, & Rowe, 1999):

- description of the process, why it needs improvement, and who is affected
- development of criteria to demonstrate that the process has improved
- timeline for meetings
- resources available
- structure of leadership (e.g., self-managed, leader directed)
- expected communication of progress, results.

d. How Do Teams Develop?

Teams develop and change over time. Tuckman (1965) described four stages of development in one popular model.

Stage 1. Forming. During the first stage, the members try to get to know each other, agree on the goal or vision, and delegate tasks. Discussions focus on how to accomplish the tasks and the information and resources needed. This is a period of testing to find out what kind of behavior is appropriate. Members tend to defer to the leader or dominant member for guidance. In this stage, team leaders need to be directive and provide role clarification.

Stage 2. Storming. This second stage is where conflict typically arises. Members try to express their individuality and resist group pressures and influence. There often are emotional responses to group demands, especially if the group is under pressure to achieve results. To prevent the group from becoming stuck at this stage, leaders need to manage the conflict—not by suppressing it, but by using it to energize the team.

Stage 3. Norming. In this stage, group members develop close ties and a strong identity with the team. There is a shift from "I" to "we" and a willingness to accept the views of others. Group members develop feelings of mutual respect, harmony, and trust. Group standards and members' roles emerge. Leaders need to challenge team members to continue to grow and guard against too much conformity to group norms.

Stage 4. Performing. In the fourth stage, the team works harmoniously toward a common goal and is very productive. The team develops a functional but flexible structure and roles are interrelated. Interpersonal conflicts are resolved and the group is highly task-oriented. In this stage, the leader needs to develop mechanisms for sharing leadership responsibilities.

Not all teams progress through these four stages and if they do, it is likely they move both forward and backward through the stages as new issues are identified. Nevertheless, the stages point to important developmental issues that have implications for team leaders and facilitators.

e. Characteristics of Effective Teams

It is widely known that teams often fail to produce the results for which they were brought together. What makes a team successful? Abundant research and practice has demonstrated that the following are important predictors of team success (see, for example, Campion, Medsker, & Higgs, 1993; George, 1995; Hackman, 1987; Katzenbach & Smith, 1994; Saunier & Hawk, 1994; Wageeman, 1997).

- competent members with technical, problem-solving, interpersonal, and organizational skills
- commitment to clear, common goal(s)
- standards of excellence
- contributions from every member
- collaborative environment (culture to support teamwork)
- leadership support

- nonhierarchical structure
- external support and recognition.

f. How Should Teams Be Evaluated?

Team performance requires formal evaluation. In general, evaluation of a team includes three criteria:

- *Productivity*—The extent to which the goals were met. Did the team accomplish what it set out to do?
- *Satisfaction of team members*—It is important that team members be able to work together in the future. To the extent that members are satisfied with the team, they will be more likely to work well together in the future.
- *Individual growth*—The extent to which individual members developed professionally by serving as a team member.

In addition to aligning the structure with QI, the leader can further enable employees to act by making certain that the organization has the right staff to deliver quality services. Two important issues come into play: skills and knowledge of staff, and how staff is deployed.

VII. Aligning Staff To Support Quality

Educating all employees at all levels of the organization is critical to the success of performance improvement. Because the most frequent cause of failure in any QI effort is uninvolved or indifferent top and middle management, it is essential that all leadership be educated from the start. Training should begin at the top and cascade down through the organization. Ultimately, senior and middle management should be part of the teaching team; this will demonstrate to employees that they are committed to TQM/QI.

A. Determining Education and Training Needs

There are many ways to determine the educational needs of QI participants (Gaucher & Coffey, 1993; Kirkpatrick, 1998; Phillips & Stone, 2002). Methods to obtain information should include

- evaluating knowledge and skills contained in the job description
- asking participants
- asking participants' supervisors
- asking others who are knowledgeable about the job (e.g., customer, peers, experts in QI)
- testing participants on their skills and knowledge
- analyzing participants' past performance appraisals.

B. Fundamentals of TQM/QI Curriculum

The curriculum should include the following elements:

- explanation of the need for organizational improvement, including individual and collective benefits of TQM/QI
- development and use of common quality language
- discussion of the organization's quality goals
- definition of the structure for TQM/QI/performance improvement
- articulation of TQM/QI philosophy
- description of the process for TQM/QI/performance improvement
- description and clarification of responsibilities
- tools and techniques to participate in teams and to manage work processes

- description of how change may affect the individual's job and work relationships.

Training should be tailored to the specific needs of each group (i.e., top management, middle management, staff). **Table 2-6** offers a comparison of topics addressed across major groups in a TQM/QI curriculum.

Table 2-6. Suggested Substantive Issues for QI Education and Training

Top Management Sequence	Middle Management Sequence	Staff Sequence
Quality as a strategic advantage	Key concepts of quality management (e.g., customer satisfaction, process management, teamwork, continuous improvement methods)	Quality awareness, definition of quality
Role of leadership in creating and sustaining quality vision	Principles of customer service	Quality participation—fundamental training in quality improvement including process improvement tools and techniques
Integrating quality values into day-to-day leadership	Managing process performance (measurement, QI tools, variation, problem solving, data collection and analysis)	Organization's mission, vision, and QI plan
Indicators for measuring and evaluating quality and organizational performance	Measurement of quality outcomes	Concepts of quality management: customer satisfaction, process improvement, teamwork, continuous improvement
Components of quality management implementation process	Management practices for building teamwork; employee involvement and recognition for customer service; team contributions for quality; team leadership skills; conflict resolution; communication skills; listening and giving feedback; accreditation standards	Promoting cooperation among co-workers within and between departments
Basic QI tools		Communication skills
Role as team leaders		Customer service
Awareness of accreditation standards		Relevant standards

C. Framework for Evaluating the Results of Training

Donald Kirkpatrick (1998), an expert in the field of training, perceives three reasons for evaluating training programs:

- to determine how to improve future training
- to determine whether the current training should be continued
- to justify the existence of the training department.

To the extent that trainers can demonstrate important outcomes from training, they will be seen as important to the TQM/QI movement and the organization itself.

Kirkpatrick (1998) suggests that there are four important levels of evaluation: reaction, learning, behavior, and results.

Reaction. This is the extent to which the participants are satisfied with training. Because negative attitudes toward the program can interfere with learning, this is an important measurement. Reactions are frequently measured at the end of the training program or soon after the program has ended through use of a questionnaire.

Learning. When participants change attitudes, improve knowledge, or increase skill as a result of the program learning has occurred. Unless one of these parameters has changed, it is unlikely that behavior will change. Learning is best measured both before and after training and, where possible, should include some type of control group to use as a basis of comparison. The type of measure used will depend upon what is being evaluated. For example, increased skill may have to be evaluated by a specialist in that particular area; whereas change in attitudes can be measured using a pre- and post-questionnaire format.

Behavior. This level refers to behavioral change as a result of the training. While positive reactions may produce a desire to change behavior and learning may give participants the skills to know how and what to change, it doesn't necessarily follow that behavior will actually change. In addition to positive reactions and learning, employees must work in a climate supportive of change and they must see some reward associated with changing their behaviors. This doesn't have to be tangible rewards; intangible rewards such as a feeling of self-achievement also are important motivators for change. The climate is heavily dependent on the support of the supervisor, further supporting the importance of all levels of management being involved in TQM/QI education and training. Ideally, behaviors are measured both before and after training, allowing ample time for behavioral change to occur. Pre- and post-training information can be collected in the form of questionnaires and interviews and should be elicited from participants as well as from those who are in a position to observe participants' behaviors (e.g., immediate supervisor, customers, peers). Some relevant behavioral changes relating to TQM/QI may include the extent to which

- department heads deploy TQM/QI concepts, methods, and tools
- senior leaders communicate the organization's values (measured by employee questionnaires and focus groups)
- leadership practices reflect employee involvement and participation.

Results. This is the last—and probably the most important—level of program evaluation. Indicators used to measure results should be tied to the driving force behind conducting training in the first place. For example, did quality of care actually improve and was this a function of TQM/QI training? Did the number of errors reported increase initially, then were overall errors reduced through organizationwide TQM/QI training? As with evaluation of behavioral changes, results evaluation should measure pre- and post-training, use a control group, allow ample time for results to be achieved, monitor results over time, and concurrently consider the cost of the training program versus the benefit. In some cases, a direct link between training and results will be difficult to prove because there are so many other factors that might influence a particular outcome. However, evidence that supports the link should be gathered.

D. Staffing Practices

There currently is great interest in the influence of staff-to-patient ratios on quality of care. While this has proved to be important, many other factors should be considered when making staffing decisions. Evidence is mixed on whether minimum staffing ratios will improve conditions for patients and for nurses (Coffman, Sergo, & Spetz, 2002). Correlations have been made, however, between errors and near errors increasing when work shifts were longer than 12 hours, when nurses worked overtime, or when they worked more than 40 hours per week (Rogers, Hwang, Scott, Aiken, & Dinges, 2004). **Figure 2-8** provides a summary of staffing factors (American Nurses Association, 1999).

Figure 2-8. Factors To Consider When Making Staffing Decisions

Patient Factors • Physical and psychosocial conditions (e.g., age, functional ability, communication skills, scheduled procedures, availability of social support)	• Number of patients for whom care is being provided
Unit Factors • Individual patient intensity • Unit-wide intensity (taking into account the heterogeneity of settings) • Variability of care	• Admissions, discharges, and transfers • Volume
Context Factors • Architecture (e.g., geographic dispersion of patients, size and layout of the individual patient rooms, arrangement of entire patient care units) • Technology (beepers, cellular phones, computers)	• Same unit or cluster of patients • Availability of support services
Staff Factors • Experience with patient population and level of experience • Learning curve for individuals and groups of nurses • Staff consistency, continuity, and cohesion	• Cross-training • Involvement in QI activities • Professional expectations

Adapted from American Nurses Association, 1999.

VIII. Aligning Rewards To Support Quality

Reward systems are critical to the success of TQM/QI. In fact, "The most damaging alignment problem to which many total quality failures have been attributed is the lack of alignment between expectations that arise from total quality change processes and reward systems" (Evans & Dean, 2003, p. 362). Rewards are important because they can serve to motivate individuals. Motivating people to provide excellent customer service is a top priority for most organizations. Therefore, before discussing rewards, it is important to understand motivation.

A. Basics of Motivation

Work motivation is the "The psychological forces that determine the *direction* of a person's behavior in an organization, a person's level of *effort*, and a person's level of *persistence*" (George & Jones, 2002, p. 181). There are many theories of motivation and each has somewhat different but complementary implications for actions managers can take to motivate employees. As such, a basic understanding of all the major theories is important. One way to view all theories is through the "motivation equation" (George & Jones, 2002). Each theory stresses different parts of the equation (see **Figure 2-9**).

Figure 2-9. Motivation Equation

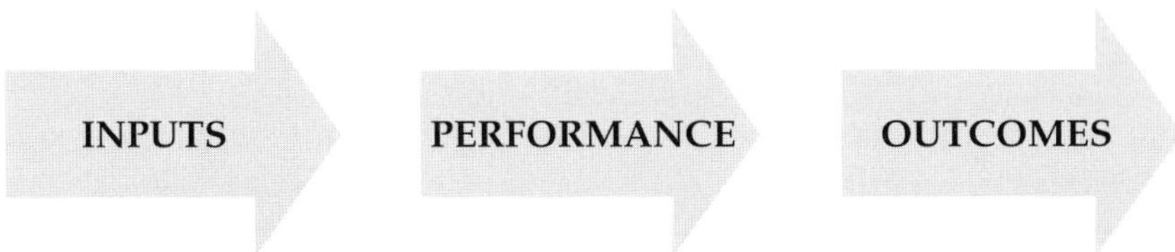

Need Theory

What *outcomes* are individuals motivated to obtain in the workplace?

Expectancy Theory

Do individuals believe that their *inputs* will result in a given level of *performance*?

Do individuals believe that *performance* at this level will lead to obtaining *outcomes* they desire?

Equity Theory

Are *outcomes* perceived as being at an appropriate level in comparison with *inputs*?

Procedural Justice

Are the *procedures* used to assess inputs and performance and to distribute outcomes perceived as fair?

Source: George & Jones. (2002). Organizational behavior. *Upper Saddle River, NJ: Prentice Hall. Reprinted with permission.*

1. Need Theories

Need theories all center on what employees are motivated to obtain from work (outcomes). Included in these theories are Maslow's hierarchy of needs, McClelland's need theory, and Hertzberg's two-factor theory.

Abraham H. Maslow's (1954) need theory was first published in 1943. Maslow, a psychologist, believed that human needs could be arranged in a hierarchy from the most basic to higher-order needs, as follows:

- physiological/survival needs (basic survival needs [food, water])
- safety/security needs (protection from harm or physical deprivation)
- belongingness/social needs (the need for interaction with others, companionship, belonging, and friendship)
- esteem/status needs (needs for recognition and appreciation)
- self-actualization needs (the need for self-fulfillment or to reach one's highest potential).

Maslow believed that basic needs had to be met before higher-order needs. For example, employees would have to meet basic survival needs (e.g., working in a safe environment) before they would focus on esteem needs. In addition, Maslow maintained that only unsatisfied needs served to motivate people; people want what they do not have.

David C. McClelland proposed a concept very similar to Maslow's, narrowing the number of needs to three types: achievement, power, and affiliation (McClelland, Atkinson, Clark, & Lowell, 1976).

Finally, Frederick Herzberg's two-factor theory classified the elements of motivation into two categories: motivators and hygiene factors (Herzberg, Maysner, & Snyderman, 1966). *Motivators* are those elements of a job that increase job satisfaction, including challenging work, achievement, recognition, growth, and advancement. *Hygiene factors*, on the other hand, did not contribute to motivation but their absence led to dissatisfaction. Hygiene factors included company policy and administrative issues such as supervision, working conditions, interpersonal relations, safety, salaries, morale, and productivity. Herzberg expanded upon Maslow's theory, making a distinction between factors that motivate versus factors that maintain motivation.

At least two managerial implications for motivation are clear from need theories:

- There are many different needs and these will not look the same among different employees.
- If employees are not motivated, managers should seek to determine what needs employees have and which are satisfied or unsatisfied.

2. Expectancy Theory

Expectancy theory is concerned with how individuals decide which behaviors to engage in and how much effort they should give to that behavior. This theory focuses on the individual's perception of effort-to-performance and performance-to-outcomes links (see Figure 2-9). Essentially, an individual asks herself, "If I work hard (effort), will I be able to perform?" Motivation is improved by strengthening that link. Managers want to be certain that employees believe that if they work hard, they will achieve high performance. Thus, providing training and education so that they have the appropriate skills to perform the work would improve motivation.

Individuals also ask themselves, "If I perform at a high level, will there be an outcome and is it something I care about?" To strengthen this performance-outcome link, managers want employees to believe that if they perform at a high level, there will be an outcome that they desire. Managers can strengthen this link by having valid performance appraisal systems that capture quality performance and also by having systems in place to reward such performance. For example, when an employee reports an adverse event, there should be an immediate outcome that is positive in the eyes of that employee.

In accordance with this theory, managers should do the following:

- Be certain employees have the necessary skills to perform well.
- Coach employees to believe that if they work hard they will be successful.
- Know what outcomes employees perceive as important (as detailed by needs theory).
- Have clear policies about what levels of performance are rewarded (result in outcomes) and which levels are not.

3. Equity Theory

Equity theory centers on the input and outcomes part of the motivation equation. The overall idea is that employees are motivated when there is fairness in the workplace. This theory contends that employees determine fairness by looking at the ratio of their inputs (work effort) to their outcomes (e.g., rewards, benefits). For example, Employee A may be motivated if she receives a financial bonus that she perceives to be equitable given her effort on the QI project. According to this theory, however, employees also compare their ratio of inputs to outcomes with that of others' inputs and outcomes. Therefore, if Employee B in the same department is awarded a larger financial bonus for the same amount of work effort, Employee A's motivation would most likely drop.

Some ways for managers to motivate employees are as follows:

- Acknowledge different performance levels with different levels of rewards.

- Periodically check employees' perceptions regarding their own input and outcomes as well as those of others.
- Know what outcomes are desirable and tie those to performance in a timely manner.

4. Procedural Justice

Procedural justice is a theory of motivation that focuses on fairness with respect to processes or procedures used to allocate outcomes. Research has demonstrated that people are more likely to see outcome allocations as fair when the following conditions exist:

- Employees have input into how decisions are made.
- There is an opportunity for performance errors to be corrected.
- Rules and policies for allocation of outcomes are applied consistently.
- Decisions are made in an unbiased manner.

B. What Do Employees Say?

There is some degree of research support for these various motivation theories. Over the past 25 years, the Gallup Organization undertook two extremely large studies. The first sought to determine, "What do the most talented employees need from their workplace?" For this part of the research, Gallup interviewed more than 1 million people who were employed across a broad range of companies, industries, and countries. This study found the "most powerful" conclusion is that retention and performance of an employee is determined "by his relationship with his immediate supervisor" (Buckingham & Coffman, 1999). So what makes a good supervisor? Gallup suggests that these data indicate that there are 12 factors critical to the retention and performance of employees:

- Do I know what is expected of me at work?
- Do I have the materials and equipment I need to do my work correctly?
- Do I have the opportunity at work to do what I do best every day?
- In the last seven days, have I received recognition or praise for doing good work?
- Does my supervisor, or someone at work, seem to care about me as a person?
- Is there someone at work who encourages my development?
- Do my opinions seem to count at work?
- Does the mission/purpose of my work organization make me feel my job is important?
- Are my coworkers committed to doing quality work?
- Do I have a best friend at work?
- In the last 6 months, has someone at work talked to me about my progress?
- This past year, have I had opportunities at work to learn and grow?

These factors clearly are consistent with the theories of motivation discussed previously.

C. Setting Up a Reward System

Given the role rewards play in employee motivation, setting up an effective reward system is important. Seven steps are fundamental to a reward system (Gaucher & Coffey, 1993):

- determine priorities and values; behaviors that will be rewarded are prioritized
- identify the criteria or milestones
- establish a budget for recognition

- determine who will be accountable for managing the recognition
- develop specific procedures and features of the rewards and recognition
- obtain feedback from employees on desired rewards and recognition
- modify program based on feedback.

The most important lesson to remember is to reward the desired behavior.

IX. Aligning Information Systems To Support Quality

Information systems play a pivotal role in TQM/QI and must also be aligned with other systems to be effective. Module One covers the role of information systems in TQM/QI/process improvement.

X. Aligning Financial Systems To Support Quality

Budgeting is a formal annual or periodic process through which financial performance goals and actual results are evaluated for the current and previous fiscal years. This allows for the development of formal goals for the next fiscal year.

A. Capital Budgeting

Capital budgeting is the process by which an organization evaluates and selects which long-term investments (or capital expenditures) it will make. These investments typically involve large initial cash outflows with the expectation that these investments will produce cash inflows in the future. Because capital assets are long-term (usually longer than 1 year), the quality of these decisions is extremely important to the organization's financial health.

Capital budgeting typically is an annual activity, but it also may be triggered by events such as requests for new programs or equipment. Capital requests are usually made formally by completion of a form such as the one shown in **Figure 2-10**. This request typically is reviewed first by financial analysts, who rate the capital expenditure proposal in terms of criteria such as feasibility, actual costs, and projected revenues. Next, the assessment is presented to senior management and members of a capital expenditures committee that comprises interdisciplinary representatives from key departments. This committee rates the proposals submitted against a variety of criteria discussed below.

Once prioritizing of proposals is completed, a final list of capital expenditures for the upcoming fiscal year is released within the organization. The capital purchases are then incorporated into the overall budgeting process. Typical capital expenditure requests from healthcare quality professionals and managers include computer equipment and software, requests for renovation and space, data purchases, and organizationwide quality initiatives or programs.

Given that resources are limited in any organization, decisions must be made as to how to select among the various proposed quality initiatives. One approach is to perform a cost-benefit analysis to support quality-related expenditures.

B. Cost-Benefit Analysis

What is cost-benefit analysis (CBA) and why is it performed? Cost-benefit analyses are performed for capital expenditure requests in order to determine the viability and broader benefits of such expenditures. This tool helps organizations to better utilize financial and human resources. For the most part, TQM/QI projects should be carried out only when the benefits exceed costs over the life of the project.

Figure 2-10. Capital and New Program Request Form

CAPITAL REQUEST ☐ NEW PROGRAM REQUEST ☐

DEPARTMENT: ______________________________

SUBMITTED BY: ____________________ TITLE: ____________________ PHONE: _______

APPROVED BY: ____________________ TITLE: ____________________ PHONE: _______

EXECUTIVE SUMMARY OF PROPOSAL:

Please explain how this proposal relates to institutional priorities according to the following criteria:

1. Mission/Business Plan:
2. Impact on Revenue:
3. Increased Efficiency?
4. Single or Multi-department Use?
5. Emergency—Service Disruption?
6. Quality of Care Enhancement?
7. Replacement or Upgrade of Equipment?

CAPITAL EQUIPMENT: CLINICAL: ☐ COMPUTER/SOFTWARE: ☐

Describe equipment: Initial Cost: ____________ (attach quote)

Maintenance Costs: ____________/yr. (quote)

Need for equipment: Emergency: ☐ Replacement: ☐ Upgrade of existing technology: ☐

Is additional space needed to accommodate? No Yes, __________sq. ft.

Are Renovations needed: No Yes __________sq. ft. of (circle one) Office Lab Clinical Care

continued

How is CBA performed? All CBAs should include a time frame, which demonstrates the costs and benefits of the project over specific periods of time. The goal is to establish a business case for the TQM/QI expenditure.

C. Establishing a Business Case for Quality-Related Expenditures

"A business case for a healthcare improvement intervention exists if the entity that invests in the intervention realizes a financial return on its investment in a reasonable time frame, using a reasonable rate of discounting. This may be

Figure 2-10. Capital and New Program Request Form *(continued)*

NEW PROGRAM REQUEST

NAME OF PROGRAM ____________________________

Why is this program needed?

What are the objectives of the program?

Will this program service new markets? If so, how wide a market geographically? What age groups?

When will this program be profitable? (Year 1, 2, 3, etc.)

Does it require new space? No Yes, __________sq. ft.

What impact will it have on the community? Healthcare providers? Employees?

Itemize all additional costs:

ITEM	INITIAL COST	ANNUAL MAINTENANCE

NEW FTEs ROLE, SALARY + FRINGE

RENOVATIONS REQUIRED

# of FTE PHYSICIANS REQUIRED

OTHER COMMENTS

realized as "bankable dollars" (profit), a reduction in losses for a given program or population, or avoided costs. In addition, a business case may exist if the investing entity believes that a positive indirect effect on organizational function and sustainability will accrue within a reasonable time frame" (Leatherman et al., 2003, p. 18).

The framework for establishing a business case for TQM/QI is set forth by Bailit and Dyer (2004). The framework centers on three broad categories for which a business case can be established:

- return on investment (ROI; the amount of financial return that an investment provides in a year)
- reduced expenditures or cost avoidance
- costs.

Investments in quality initiatives may be undertaken by a healthcare facility because of

- regulatory or contractual requirements, or performance incentives (or disincentives) offered to the organization by a variety of groups such as purchasers or providers
- alignment with explicit performance incentives (e.g., pay-for-performance initiative)
- a strategic advantage over competition by bolstering image and reputation or by marketing a particular product (development of brand identity).

Although strategic considerations typically focus staff toward the external world, organizations also must consider the nature of the internal environment when deciding about funding quality initiatives. Two important issues are relevance to the organization's mission and relevance to its culture.

XI. Organizational Renewal To Support Quality

Two important features of organizational renewal are change and innovation; these topics are considered in detail in Module Four. Another feature of renewal concerns organizational learning.

TQM/QI cannot occur without learning. If quality improvement is an ongoing process, then organizations must continuously learn. Organizational learning is a concept developed by Peter Senge (1990) to describe organizations "skilled at creating, acquiring and transferring knowledge, and at modifying its behavior to reflect new knowledge and insights" (Garvin, 1993, p. 80). According to Garvin, learning organizations are adept at performing five critical activities:

- solving problems systematically
- experimenting with new approaches
- learning from their own past experiences
- learning from the past experiences and best practices of others
- transferring knowledge quickly and efficiently throughout the organization.

Kline and Saunders (1998) suggest that organizations can set the stage for learning through adherence to a number of principles, including the following:

- Encourage self-directed behavior so that people can learn to help themselves. Teach individuals the process of self-evaluation. Help them to find ways to structure their own learning opportunities beyond the formal classroom.
- Realign structures and systems to meet the changing needs of the organization. For example, General Electric's former CEO Jack Welch coined the term "boundarylessness" to convey the need to go beyond one's own group so that new ideas could be stimulated (e.g., reducing "silo thinking"). Leaders need to provide opportunities to stimulate employee ideas (e.g., conferences, working with other departments).
- Foster a culture that supports personal growth and self-esteem. Celebrate learning as an important goal in itself and one that all organizational participants should aspire to regardless of their place in the hierarchy.
- Recognize that mistakes are a necessary part of learning and growing. Make it "safe" to make mistakes as people experiment with new ideas.

Although creating a culture of learning will take time and persistence, given the rising complexity of the healthcare system and the enormity of the problems, establishing learning as a core value will be critical to meeting the healthcare improvement aims set forth by the IOM.

XII. Performance Assessment: Measuring Results

A. Overview of Performance Improvement

Definitions and requirements for quality in healthcare have evolved over the past decades. Early in the 1950s, quality care review was conducted exclusively by individual physicians utilizing an unstructured and subjective process, which relied on the practitioner's knowledge and experiences. Between 1950 and 1960, the responsibility for quality of care expanded *beyond the physician* to include both the hospital and the board of directors. Two significant legal decisions marked this transition period:

- *Bing v. Thunig* (1957). In this case, the New York Court of Appeals ruled that the doctrine of charitable immunity no longer applied to hospitals; hospitals are liable for patient injuries sustained through negligence of employees.
- *Darling v. Charleston Community Memorial Hospital* (1965). In this important corporate negligence case, the court ruled that the hospital had a legal responsibility to protect a patient from harm by others by overseeing the quality of patient care.

B. Retrospective Audits

A shift from physician review to medical audits occurred in 1955. Medical audits included a systematic procedure using objective, valid criteria with an orientation on outcomes. In 1966 there was a major change whereby the Joint Commission on Accreditation of Hospitals (as it was called then) focused on optimal, not minimal, standards of care. In 1975, the Joint Commission published the quality of professional services standards, requiring hospitals to demonstrate optimal care using valid and reliable measures. While *optimal* was never defined, this new focus led to one-time audits of care, known as performance evaluation programs audits.

C. Quality Assurance

Audits soon led to a preoccupation with meeting audit number requirements. As a result, in 1980 the Joint Commission developed the first quality assurance standards requiring a problem-focused approach to measuring quality. This approach required organizations to identify and monitor problem areas.

The combined strengths of criteria-based audits and the epidemiological approach used in infection control in the 1980s resulted in a new focus on systematic monitoring and evaluation in 1985. From this, a 10-step process for quality improvement evolved in 1986 requiring organizations to evaluate important aspects of care and then use the results to identify opportunities for improvement.

D. Quality Improvement Method

By the early 1990s TQM/QI methodologies were becoming commonplace in healthcare facilities.

In 1994, the Joint Commission introduced the new standards on improving organizational performance, requiring a collaborative culture that focuses on processes by understanding how customers define quality, how processes work, and understanding the importance of reducing variation in those processes (Joint Commission, 1994). This represents a shift in focus from the performance of individuals to the performance of the organization's systems and processes. There is no longer any department-specific review (e.g., no ancillary services review for performance improvement); performance improvement is reviewed for the entire organization (Joint Commission, 1994). The new standards also required a shift from improving only clinical quality to improving nonclinical care, value, and patient satisfaction.

The following discussion on performance management centers on the organizational level and in the context of meeting the organization's strategic goals and objectives.

E. Performance Management

Performance management has been defined as: "The use of performance management information to effect positive change in organizational culture, systems and processes, by helping to set agreed-upon performance goals, allocating and prioritizing resources, informing managers to either confirm or change current policy or program direction to meet those goals, and sharing results of performance in pursuing those goals" (Office of Procurement and Assistance Management, 2005, p. 7). The goal of a performance management system is to make certain that the vision of the organization is being met by defining and measuring outcomes reflected in that vision.

Although there is a variety of quality performance programs, including the Baldrige National Quality Program and the European Foundation for Quality Management, a significant percentage of government agencies and *Fortune* 1000 companies presently use the balanced scorecard (BSC) as an approach to performance management. BSCs are completely compatible with other quality performance programs but go beyond such programs by embedding QI within the strategic framework of the organization (Kaplan & Bower, 2001).

The BSC was developed by Drs. David Norton and Robert Kaplan in the early 1990s. The basic idea is that performance measures should provide a comprehensive view of organizational performance and not be overly dependent on a few choice indicators. Unlike other performance models, the BSC helps organizations to better link long-term strategy with short-term activities (Kaplan & Norton, 1996).

The BSC approach views the organization from four different perspectives or categories: financial ("How do we look to providers of financial resources?"), customer ("How do our customers see us?"), internal business processes ("At what must we excel?"), and learning and growth ("Can we continue to improve and create value for customers?"). Answers to these questions influence the nature of the strategic goals and objectives that are set and, ultimately, what performance measures are used. The critical aspect of performance indicators is that they must reflect the organization's strategic goals and objectives.

There are likely to be several strategic objectives corresponding to each of the four perspectives. Each of these objectives should have at least one measure, and the principles as described in Module One regarding measure precision, reliability, validity, and mixture of qualitative and quantitative all hold true here. In addition, data can be collected from a variety of means (e.g., surveys, focus groups, patient chart reviews).

Kelly (2003) suggests that development and use of different types of measures (i.e., structure, process, and outcomes) within each of the categories is an important approach. Examples of the four categories and measures within the context of the strategic goals and objectives discussed earlier (see Table 2-3) are presented next.

The foundation for an organization's strategic success begins with its people, who must be willing to *learn and grow*. To meet the changing needs of customers they must, for example, be able to learn new technology and acquire new skills in order to take on new responsibilities. For the strategic goal, "Develop state-of-the-art program for breast cancer detection and treatment" (Table 2-3), measures could include

- structure: quantity of imaging equipment
- process: number of patients diagnosed with imaging technology
- outcome: higher percentage of early diagnoses, due to use of imaging technology.

It is necessary to monitor and improve key *processes* so that employees are able to convert learning and growth into products and services—quality outcomes. "To be recognized as one of the top providers in the community" was another strategic goal (Table 2-3). Measures could include

- structure: nurse to patient ratio
- process: governance model used by the organization
- outcomes: decreased turnover of nursing staff.

Customer satisfaction is important, and high-quality outcomes, including patient education, will improve satisfaction. The strategic goals (Table 2-3) included "Establish outreach program for management of chronic illnesses." Measures associated with this objective could include

- structure: number of staff educated on outreach
- process: hours of outreach education by staff
- outcomes: new referrals.

Depending on the nature of the organization, the *financial* perspective can cover a wide range of outcomes (e.g., efficiency, effectiveness, profits). High-quality care should have a positive effect on customer loyalty. For the goal of being a top provider in the community, measures could include

- structure: positive image campaign
- process: partnering with key physician groups
- outcomes: increased market share.

Just as different organizational levels and units develop goals and objectives based on corporate strategy, different levels and units also can utilize BSC. Also, note that for the same strategic goal (e.g., top provider in community) there are several measures of performance across different perspectives.

Note how the four perspectives are interrelated. For example, competent employees give good care, resulting in satisfied and loyal customers, resulting in a greater market share. The complexity of performance measures is a good match for the complexity of healthcare organizations.

References

American Nurses Association. (1999). *Principles for nurse staffing*. Retrieved May 6, 2005, from http://www.nursingworld.org/readroom/stffprnc.htm

Anderson, R.A., & McDaniel, R.R. (2000). Managing health care organizations: Where professionalism meets complex science. *Health Care Management Review, 25*(1), 83–92.

Axtell, R.N., & Eckholdt, S.L. (1992). "Organizational Systems Design: Enriching Lives by Creating Self-Designing Organizations" Workshop. Presented by the Alliance of Organizational System Designers, Snowbird, Utah, September 23–25.

Bailit, M., & Dyer, M. (2004). *Beyond bankable dollars: Establishing a business case for improving healthcare*. New York: The Commonwealth Fund.

Baird, K. (2000). *Customer service in health care: A grassroots approach to creating a culture of service excellence*. San Francisco: Jossey-Bass.

Baldrige National Quality Program. (2005). *Health care criteria for performance excellence*, p. 11. Retrieved May 31, 2005, from www.quality.nist.gov/HealthCare_Criteria.htm

Begun, J., Zimmerman, B., & Dooley, K. (2003). Health care organizations as complex Adaptive Systems, in S. Mick, & M. Wyttenbach (Eds). *Advances in health care organization theory* (pp. 253–258). San Francisco: Jossey-Bass.

Buckingham, M., & Coffman, C. (1999). *First, break all the rules: What the world's greatest managers do differently*. New York: Simon & Schuster.

Campion, M.A., Medsker, G.J., & Higgs, C. A. (1993). Relations between work group characteristics and effectiveness: Implications for designing effective work groups. *Personnel Psychology, 46*, 823–850.

Coffman, J.M., Sergo, J.A., & Spetz, J. (2002). Minimum nurse-to-patient ratios in acute care hospitals in California. *Health Affairs, 21*(s). 53-64.

Committee on Quality of Health Care in America, Institute of Medicine. (2001). *Crossing the quality chasm: A new health system for the 21st century*. Washington, DC: National Academies Press.

Deming, W.E. (1986). *Out of the crisis*. Cambridge, MA: MIT Center for Advanced Engineering Studies.

Donabedian, A. (1980). *The definition of quality and approaches to its assessment*. Ann Arbor, MI: Health Administration Press.

Dunham, R.B., & Pierce, J.L. (1989). *Management*. Glenview, IL: Scott Foresman and Company.

Evans, J.R., & Dean, J.W. (2003). *Total quality: Management, organization and strategy* (3rd Ed.). Mason, OH: Thomson South-Western.

Fisher, S., & Samways, M. (1985). *Write better behavioral objectives*. (Infoline #5). Alexandria, VA: American Society for Training and Development.

Garvin, D.A. (1993). Building a learning organization. *Harvard Business Review, 71*, 78–91.

Gaucher, E.J., & Coffey, R.J. (1993). *Total quality in healthcare: From theory to practice*. San Francisco: Jossey-Bass Publishers.

George, J.M. (1995). Leader positive mood and group performance: The case of customer service. *Journal of Applied Social Psychology, 25*, 778–794.

George, J.M., & Jones, G.R. (2002). *Organizational behavior* (3rd ed.). Upper Saddle River, NJ: Prentice Hall.

Ginter, P.M., Swayne, L.E., & Duncan, W.J. (2002). *Strategic management of health care organizations* (4th ed.). Oxford, UK: Blackwell Publishers.

Greenberg, J., & Baron, R.A. (2003). *Behavior in organizations* (8th ed.). Upper Saddle River, NJ: Prentice Hall.

Hackman, J.R. (1987). The design of work teams. In J.W. Lorsch (Ed.), *Handbook of organizational behavior*. Upper Saddle River, NJ: Prentice Hall.

Herzberg, F., Maysner, B., & Snyderman, B. (1966). *Works and the nature of man*. New York: John Wiley & Sons, Inc.

House, C., & Price, R. (1991). The return map: Track product teams. *Harvard Business Review, 60*(1), 93.

Joint Commission on Accreditation of Healthcare Organizations. (1994). *Framework for improving performance: A guide for nurses*. Oakbrook Terrace, IL: Author.

Juran, J.M. (1989). *Juran on leadership for quality: An executive handbook*. New York: The Free Press.

Kaplan, R., & Bower, M. (2001). The balanced scorecard and quality programs. *Balanced Scorecard Report* (newsletter), Mar 15, 3–6. Cambridge, MA: Harvard Business School Publishing.

Kaplan, R., & Norton, D. (1996). Using the balanced scorecard as a strategic management system. *Harvard Business Review, 74*, 75–85.

Katzenbach, J.R., & Smith, D.K. (1994). *The wisdom of teams: Creating the high-performance organization*. Boston, MA: Harvard Business School Press.

Kavaler, F., & Spiegel, A. (1997). *Risk management in health care institutions: A strategic approach*. Sudbury, MA: Jones & Bartlett Publishers.

Kelly, D. (2003). *Applying quality management in healthcare: A process for improvement*. Chicago: Health Administration Press.

Kirkpatrick, D.L. (1998). *Evaluating training programs* (2nd ed.). San Francisco: Berrett-Koehler Publishers, Inc.

Kline, P., & Saunders, B. (1998). *Ten steps to a learning organization* (2nd ed.). Arlington, VA: Great Ocean Publishers.

Kotter, J.P. (1990). What leaders really do. *Harvard Business Review, 68*, 103–111.

Kouzes, J.M., & Posner, B.Z. (2002). *Leadership: The challenge*. San Francisco: Jossey-Bass—A Wiley Imprint.

Kuhn, A.M., & Youngberg, B.J. (2002). The need for risk management to evolve to assure a culture of safety. *Quality and Safety in Health Care, 11*, 158–162.

Leatherman, S., Berwick, D., Illes, D., Lewin, L., Davidoff, F., Nolan, T., et al. (2003). The business case for quality: Case studies and an analysis. *Health Affairs, 22*(2), 17–30.

Luecke, R. (2004). *Creating teams with an edge: The complete skill set to build powerful and influential teams*. Harvard Business Essentials Series. Boston: Harvard Business School Press.

Luthans, F., Hodgetts, R., & Thompson, K. (1990). *Social issues in business: Strategic and public policy perspectives* (6th ed.). Upper Saddle River, NJ: Prentice Hall Inc.

Maslow, A. (1954). *Motivation and personality*. New York: Harper and Row.

McClelland, D.C., Atkinson, J.W., Clark, R.A., & Lowell, E.L. (1976). *The achievement motive*. New York: Irvington.

Merriam-Webster's collegiate dictionary (10th ed.). (1994). Springfield, MA: Merriam-Webster.

Milliman, W., & Robertson, S. (Eds.). (1995). *Healthcare management guidelines*. Seattle: Milliman & Robertson, Inc.

National Association for Healthcare Quality (NAHQ). (1998). *NAHQ guide to quality management* (8th ed.). Glenview, IL: Author.

Office of Procurement and Assistance Management. (2005). *Balanced Scorecard Performance measurement and performance management program*, p. 7. Retrieved June 7, 2005, from http://professionals.pr.doe.gov/ma5/MA-5Web.nsf/Business/Balanced+Scorecard?OpenDocument

Orlikoff, J.E. (1990). *Quality from the top: Working with hospital governing boards to assure quality care*. Chicago: Pluribus Press.

Peters, T., & Waterman, R. (1982). *In search of excellence*. New York: Harper & Row.

Phillips J., & Stone, R. (2002). *How to measure training results: A practical guide to tracking the six key indicators*. New York: McGraw-Hill.

Porter-O'Grady, T., Hawkins, M.A., & Parker, M.L. (1997). *Whole-systems shared governance: Architecture for integration*. Gaithersburg, MD: Aspen Publishers.

Robbins, S.P. (2001). *Organizational behavior* (8th Ed.) Upper Saddle River, NJ: Prentice Hall.

Rogers, A.E., Hwang, W.T., Scott, L.D., Aiken, L.H. & Diages, D.F. (2004). The working hours of hospital staff nurses and patient safety. *Health Affairs, 23*(4), 202-212.

Rokeach, M. (1973). *The nature of human values*. New York: Free Press.

Saunier, A.M., & Hawk, E.J. (1994). Realizing the potential of teams through team-based rewards. *Compensation & Benefits Review, 10*, 24–33.

Schein, E.H. (1992). *Organizational culture and leadership: A dynamic view* (2nd ed.). San Francisco: Jossey-Bass.

Schneider, B. (Ed.). (1990). *Organizational culture and climate*. San Francisco: Jossey-Bass.

Schwarz, M., Landis, S., & Rowe, J. (1999, April). A team approach to quality improvement. *Family Practice Management*, 6, 25–31.

Senge, P.M. (1990). *The fifth discipline: The art & practice of the learning organization*. New York: Doubleday Publishing.

Shortell, S.M., Morrison, E., & Robbins, S. (1985). Strategy-making in health care organizations: A framework and agenda for research. *Medical Care Review, 2*, 219–266.

Siehl, L., & Martin, J. (1981). *Learning organizational culture*. [Working paper]. Palo Alto, CA: Stanford University, Graduate School of Business.

SSM Health Care. *SSM Health Care home page*. Retrieved May 5, 2005, from http://www.ssmhc.com/internet/home/ssmcorp.nsf

Stamatis, D.H. (1996). *Total quality management in healthcare: Implementation strategies for optimum results*. Chicago: Irwin Publishing.

Thompson, A. A, Jr., & Strickland, A.J., III. (1996). *Strategic management: Concepts and cases*, 9th ed. Boston, MA: Irwin McGraw-Hill.

Thompson, L. (2000). *Making the team: A guide for managers*. Upper Saddle River, NJ: Prentice Hall.

Tuckman, W. (1965). Developmental sequence in small groups. *Psychological Bulletin, 63*, 384–399.

Wageman, R. (1997). Critical success factors for creating superb self-managing teams. *Organizational Dynamics, 26*, 49–61.

Suggested Reading

Covey, S.R. (1989). *The seven habits of highly effective people.* New York: Simon and Schuster.

Dolence, M.G., Rowley, D.J., & Lujar, H.D. (1997). *Working toward strategic change: A step-by-step guide to the planning process.* San Francisco: Jossey-Bass.

Fottler, M.D., Ford, R.C., & Heaton, C.P. (2002). *Achieving service excellence: Strategies for healthcare.* Chicago: Health Administration Press.

Fried, B.J., & Johnson, J.A. (2001). *Human resources in healthcare: Managing for success.* Chicago: Health Administration Press.

Gaucher, E.J., & Coffey, R.J. (2000). *Breakthrough performance: Accelerating the transformation of health care organizations.* San Francisco: Jossey-Bass Publishers.

Griffith, J.R., & White, K.R. (2003). *Thinking forward: Six strategies for highly successful organizations.* Chicago: Health Administration Press.

Hadelman, J. (2000). *The impact of strategic healthcare leadership: Top ten leadership trends in health care in the 21st century.* Oak Brook, IL: Witt/Kieffer.

Helmrich, R.L., & Merritt, A.C. (1998). *Culture at work in aviation and medicine.* Aldershot, UK, Ashgate Publishing Limited.

Hess, R.G. (2004). From bedside to boardroom–Nursing shared governance. *Online Journal of Issues in Nursing*, 9(1), January, 31. Retrieved May 5, 2005, from http://www.nursingworld.org/ojin/topic23/tpc23_1.htm

Horak, B.J. (1999). *Strategic planning in healthcare: Building a quality-based plan step-by-step.* Portland, OR: Book News, Inc.

Katzenbach, J.R. (1998). *Teams at the top.* Cambridge, MA: Harvard Business School Press.

Kerr, S. (1995). On the folly of rewarding A, while hoping for B. *Academy of Management Executive, 9*(1), 7–14.

Kotter, J.P. (1995). Why transformation efforts fail. *Harvard Business Review,* March-April, 59–67.

Kotter, J.P. (1996). *Leading change.* Boston: Harvard Business School Press.

Kouzes, J.M., & Posner, B.Z. (1995). *Leadership challenge: How to get extraordinary things done in organizations.* San Francisco: Jossey-Bass Publishers.

McLaughlin, C.P., & Kaluzny, A.D. (1999). *Continuous quality improvement in health care: Theory, implementation, and applications* (2nd ed.). Gaithersburg, MD: Aspen Publishers.

Pointer, D.D., & Ewell, C.M. (1995). Really governing: What type of work should boards be doing? *Journal of Healthcare Management, 40*(3), 315–332.

Quinn, R.E. (1996). *Deep change: Discovering the leader within.* San Francisco: Jossey-Bass Publishers.

Quinn, R.E., & Camerson, K.S. (1999). *Diagnosing and changing organizational culture.* Reading, MA: Addison-Wesley.

Roberts, K.H., & Bea, R. (2001). Must accidents happen? Lessons from high-reliability organizations. *Academy of Management Executive, 15*, 70–78.

Schmele, J.A. (1996). *Quality management in nursing and health care.* Albany, NY: Delmar Publishers.

Shortell, S.M., & Kaluzny, A.D. (2005). *Health care management: Organization design and behavior*. Albany, NY: Delmar Thomson Learning Publishers.

Tyler, J.L., & Biggs, E. (2001). *Practical governance.* Chicago: Health Administration Press.

Whetten, D.A., & Cameron, K.S. (1995). *Developing management skills* (3rd ed.) New York: HarperCollins College Publishers.

SOLUTIONS

MODULE THREE

Continuous Readiness

Diane Brown, PhD MSN RN CPHQ FNAHQ

I. Context of Continuous Readiness

Reflect on experiences with accreditation surveys. Were there ramp-up activities in the months prior to the survey to ensure compliance? Did this require tremendous additional resources in order to be successful, such as additional time, energy, people (including internal and external consultants), extra meetings, new work, and copy or production costs? Was the organization's approach just-in-time training for staff and action? Was there tremendous relief when it was over and it was promised that the next 2- or 3-year cycle would be different? Was the organization's culture one in which a 2- or 3-year hiatus was expected until the next ramp-up? Was it difficult to get leadership's attention for identified compliance issues after survey because the last survey had been successful? Were there unplanned surveys or regulatory visits that did not go well and then required additional resources to regain compliance? Have you described your job as "crisis management"?

Many of the above scenarios will be familiar to most healthcare quality professionals. After all, we have practiced continuous improvement by solving the same problems over and over again. The image described above defines what a culture of continuous readiness *is not* and prepares healthcare quality professionals to begin a journey to understand and deploy what it really is.

To begin this journey of understanding and creating a culture of continuous readiness, it is useful to first understand the concept itself. The mode of compliance readiness on a continuous basis might best be understood by examining the words individually. *Culture* is defined as the set of shared attitudes, values, goals, and practices that characterizes a company or corporation (Merriam-Webster Online Dictionary, 2004). *Continuous* is defined as uninterrupted extension in sequence or an uninterrupted flow; *readiness* is defined as being prepared mentally or physically for some experience or action, immediately available, or ready for immediate use (Merriam-Webster). The outcome of these activities is the demonstration of *compliance*, which is defined as conformity in fulfilling official requirements.

With these definitions, a culture of continuous readiness is a company or corporate attitude and value; this is demonstrated throughout the organization in goals and practices of an uninterrupted state of mental preparedness and by being immediately physically ready or available to demonstrate compliance. Given the current culture of healthcare and public expectations for safe patient care, "survey readiness" is not a central focus in this definition as each patient, rather than each survey, deserves continuous compliance. Compliance can be demonstrated in a variety of ways and is not limited to survey processes through regulatory or accrediting agency visits. However, agency visits are one of the most visible (and stressful) mechanisms for demonstrating compliance.

II. Surveys Requiring Continuous Readiness

The concept of continuous readiness applies to a variety of types of surveys by numerous governmental and private organizations. An example of a survey within healthcare facilities would be a corporate survey that is conducted by internal corporate consultants to evaluate compliance with company regulations and policies or to conduct oversight for boards of directors. There are surveys conducted by those who pay for health services to ensure compliance with any conditions of participation. There are regulatory agencies, such as state departments of health services, which conduct licensing surveys or investigate complaints. And there are a variety of accreditation surveys.

The largest health insurer or payer for healthcare services in the United States is the Centers for Medicare & Medicaid Services (CMS). CMS surveys and certifies healthcare facilities to determine compliance with CMS quality standards and to investigate complaints from the public. CMS administers the Medicare program and works in partnership with all 50 states to administer Medicaid and the State Children's Health Insurance Program (www.cms.hhs.gov). These programs account for 45% of the nation's healthcare dollars, covering 83 million beneficiaries (or more than one in four Americans). Medicare is a social insurance program financed by payroll taxes from workers and their employers, beneficiary premium payments, and general federal revenues, whereas Medicaid provides medical care for low-income and uninsured individuals. CMS also contracts with independent medical organizations to ensure that medical care paid for by Medicare meets professionally recognized standards of healthcare. CMS measures and works to improve outcomes of care by educating healthcare providers about quality improvement (QI) opportunities, and educating beneficiaries to make good healthcare choices by providing comparative quality information for consumers on its Web site.

Individual states have Departments of Health Services (DHS), which have a variety of programs (including licensing and certification programs) that operate licensing and enforcement programs in accordance with state licensing and federal certification requirements. These programs also may ensure quality of care through a variety of other activities as well as management of state Medicaid programs. As an example, the California DHS has required QI activities, policy, partnerships with public and private healthcare providers, and programs that promote the use of practice guidelines (www.dhs.ca.gov).

An example of federal certification requirements is CMS's regulation of all laboratory testing performed on human subjects through the Clinical Laboratory Improvement Amendments (CLIA; www.cms.hhs.gov/clia). The division of laboratory services, within the survey and certification group, is responsible for implementing the CLIA program. All clinical laboratories must be certified to receive Medicare or Medicaid payments. CLIA has a list of CMS-approved accrediting organizations that may perform laboratory inspections; its requirements are deemed as being equivalent to or more stringent than CMS's regulatory requirements (CMS accepts the accrediting organization's inspection in lieu of its own inspection). Organizations accredited by CLIA include the American Association of Blood Banks, the American Osteopathic Association, the American Society of Histocompatibility and Immunogenetics, the College of American Pathologists, the Commission of Office Laboratory Accreditation (COLA), and the Joint Commission on Accreditation of Healthcare Organizations.

Accreditation provides an external "seal of approval." Usually a voluntary process, accreditation indicates that a facility or service has passed a standardized objective review process (usually an on-site survey) conducted by an impartial organization and that it meets guidelines or nationally/internationally recognized performance standards. Some states accept accreditation to meet regulatory requirements for state licensure. Based on this accreditation, a hospital, for example, would not routinely be surveyed by state agencies to determine compliance with CMS conditions of participation.

The accreditation cycle varies with each organization, but many are 2- or 3-year cycles. Cycles begin with an application requesting an accreditation review. The accrediting organization reviews the application to determine the scope of the review by evaluating the size of the organization, services to be reviewed, and types of agencies involved. An inspection or survey team is assigned, and a date for the survey is determined with the applicant. Documents may be requested in advance of the on-site survey and may be assembled for on-site review or submitted in advance either electronically or via mail systems. The on-site review is conducted by professionals with credentials in the field of review. The length of the review is dependent on the size of the organization and the complexity of services offered. Most reviews conclude with a summation conference by the review team to inform leadership of compliance findings and accreditation scoring. A report of the findings may be left upon the review team's exit or provided to the organization at a later date. Any deficiencies or requirements for improvement must be corrected and documentation submitted to the accrediting organization within predetermined timeframes. Accreditation status often is listed on the accreditation organization's Web site as public information and may include additional performance data. Several accreditation organizations require a periodic self-assessment or performance review between accreditation surveys to help ensure continuous compliance. Fees associated with accreditation may be annual payments, submitted with applications, or paid after on-site inspections. Because these fees can be substantial, they must be included in operating budgets.

The following accreditation organizations in the United States represent only a sampling of those available.

National Committee for Quality Assurance. NCQA evaluates the quality of care and service provided by healthcare organizations. NCQA assesses organization performance against standards for care and service delivery, including HEDIS and through a member satisfaction survey. NCQA accredits the following types of programs: managed care organizations; managed behavioral healthcare organizations; preferred provider organizations; disease management; new health plans; VA human research protection accreditation program; partnership for human research protection accreditation program; and interactive survey system overview. NCQA certifies the following programs: credentials verification organization; physician organization; utilization management and credentialing; disease management; privacy certification for business associates; and interactive survey system overview. The NCQA Web site (www.ncqa.org) provides information about its programs, publications, resources, and health plan report card data for purchasers and consumers.

Joint Commission on Accreditation of Healthcare Organizations. The Joint Commission aims to improve the safety of care using accreditation and certification as risk-reduction activities; compliance with standards is intended to reduce the risk of adverse outcomes. The Joint Commission accredits the following types of healthcare organizations: hospitals; healthcare networks (managed care plans, preferred provider organizations, integrated delivery networks, and managed behavioral health); home healthcare organizations (home health, hospice, home infusion, durable medical equipment, personal care and support); nursing homes and other long-term care facilities; assisted living facilities; behavioral healthcare organizations; ambulatory care providers; and clinical laboratories. It certifies the following types of programs: disease-specific care, healthcare staffing, lung volume reduction surgery, and left ventricular assist device implantation. The organization's Web site (www.jcaho.org) provides information to consumers, such as quality report cards on accredited organizations, and information for professionals, such as education and other resources.

Utilization Review Accreditation Commission. The commission shortened its name to the acronym "URAC" when its accreditation programs grew to include other types of organizations such as health plans and PPOs. URAC also uses a second corporate name, the American Accreditation HealthCare Commission. The following accreditation programs are offered: case management, claims processing, consumer-directed health, core accreditation, credentials verification organization, disease management, health call center, health network, health plan, health provider credentialing, health utilization management, health Web site, Health Insurance Portability and Accountability Act (HIPAA) privacy, HIPAA security, independent review, and workers' compensation utilization management. The URAC Web site (www.urac.org) offers consumer information, information about programs and services, education, publications, and other resource information.

Healthcare Facilities Accreditation Program. The American Osteopathic Association's (AOA) HFAP accredits acute-care hospitals, hospital laboratories, ambulatory care/surgery, mental health, substance abuse, and physical rehabilitation medicine facilities. The AOA Web site (www.osteopathic.org) provides information about osteopathic medicine, policies, community resources, accreditation, and a listing of accredited health facilities.

Commission on Accreditation of Rehabilitation Facilities. CARF's mission is to promote the quality, value, and optimal outcomes of services through a consultative accreditation process. The CARF Web site (www.carf.org) provides information to consumers about accreditation and assistance in finding an accredited provider; for professionals, there is information about available publications and educational opportunities.

Commission of Office Laboratory Accreditation. COLA was founded in 1998 as a private alternative to help laboratories stay in compliance with CLIA. COLA accredits physician office laboratories in compliance with CLIA, hospitals, and independent laboratories. The COLA Web site (www.cola.org) provides information about laboratory accreditation programs, educational opportunities, manufacturers and associations, and other resources.

College of American Pathologists. In addition to general laboratory accreditation, CAP also provides specialty programs for reproductive laboratories and forensic urine drug-testing programs. The CAP Web site (www.cap.org) provides organizational information, education, news, and links to related sites. It also provides checklists for the most frequently cited deficiencies in laboratory accreditation inspections, organized into 20 topics. The checklists provide evaluation questions related to specific compliance standards to assist laboratories with self-assessment.

III. Creating a Culture of Continuous Readiness

Given the definition of continuous readiness, it is helpful to examine a framework for understanding processes to achieve this culture by understanding how to lead change within complex organizations or systems.

A. Healthcare Organizations as Complex Adaptive Systems

Complexity science is an emerging field that has recently been applied to healthcare as a different way to understand complex human organizations. It provides a useful alternative to the machine metaphor, which was first used by Newton to make sense of the world (Zimmerman, Lindberg, & Plsek, 2001). A Newtonian model of a machine suggests that the parts can explain the whole, whereas complexity science suggests that the whole is not the sum of the parts. Rather than attempting to understand organizations by examination of the parts in a linear model, it is an acknowledgment that groups of people create outcomes and effects that are far greater than would have been predicted by summing up the resources and skills available within the group. Three concepts—independent agents, distributed control, and nonlinearity—create conditions for perpetual innovation as the complex adaptive systems learn new strategies from experience. The history of where they have been will shape their future. These concepts resonate with quality professionals while reflecting on previous organizational experiences.

Processes or systems can be classified as "simple," "complicated," or "complex" (Plsek, 2004). Simple processes allow people to follow a prescribed procedure to get the same results every time; for example, cooking with a recipe that has been tested ensures replicability without particular expertise. An example in the quality field might be running preprogrammed or automated reports. Complicated processes require a high level of expertise in many specialized fields and coordination to achieve a high degree of certainty of the outcome; for example, launching a moon rocket where the formulas are critical and necessary, and one successful launch increases the likelihood that the next launch will occur as planned. Complex processes have uncertain outcomes even when formulas or prescriptive procedures have been developed and expertise is available; for example, raising one child successfully gives no assurance of success with the next child. An example in healthcare might be staffing a nursing unit for the next shift. Although it has long been recognized that organizations are complicated, there has not been further differentiation to understand them as complex organizations nor an appreciation for how that dynamic affects healthcare quality programs.

Healthcare organizations are complex adaptive systems (CAS). This means that as a system of interdependent things (agents that can be people, departments, etc.) there are a great number of connections between a wide variety of elements in addition to the ability to learn from experience (Zimmerman et al., 2001). The "parts" have the ability to respond in different and unpredictable ways, which can manifest as innovation and creative behavior or as errors (Plsek, 2001). Each agent (person or department) acts based on local knowledge and conditions, and their actions are not controlled by a central body; control is distributed throughout the CAS system rather than centralized. Centralized control slows down the capacity to react and adapt. Consider that in many healthcare delivery systems, operations are 24 hours a day, 7 days a week, whereas traditional executives (central body) may work only Monday through Friday during normal business hours. CAS also are "nested" in other CAS: for example, a physician is a CAS but also an agent in the department; the department is a CAS and an agent in the hospital; the hospital is a CAS and an agent in a multisystem organization; and the organization is a CAS and an agent in the healthcare system. The entire system emerges from a pattern of interactions.

CAS use variety or diversity as a source of information, which is seen as a key source of sustainability—the key to innovation and long-term viability (Zimmerman et al., 2001). Relationships between individuals are a critical component of the CAS model. Using team sports as an analogy, a team with the best individual players can lose to a team of poorer players when the second team focuses on creating outcomes that are beyond the talents or capabilities of an individual. Team members on healthcare team improvement projects who present diverse thinking styles are more likely to produce more information to solve problems or improve care.

The outcomes of a CAS emerge from a process of self-organization, which emerges from interrelationships (Zimmerman et al., 2001). How the system will evolve is therefore unpredictable. The co-evolution of a CAS and its environment is difficult to map because it is not linear. The size of the outcome may not be correlated to the size of the input. We all can relate to experiences in which a small effort has resulted in huge change and, conversely, to situations in which a huge effort has resulted in little, if any, demonstrable change. For example, a big push after a retreat or strategic planning session may not result in change. In contrast, one small push to the system, such as a piece of gossip, may create radical or rapid change in an organization.

CAS are naturally drawn to attractors, which is a pattern or area that draws the energy of the system to it (Zimmerman et al., 2001). Using this concept flips change management perspectives from overcoming resistance to change, to using the natural energy of the system rather than to fight against it. The study of CASs in nature and applying this to organizations has provided insight into how change occurs in human systems (Plsek & Kilo, 1999). A key finding has been that change is occurring naturally within the existing system. Reflection on how healthcare has changed over the years demonstrates that we have naturally adopted many new procedures, medications, systems, and technologies. Change is not so much about overcoming resistance as it is about creating attraction. What has been labeled "resistance" is really an attraction to factors in the current system that we might not fully understand or appreciate. Resistance is a natural, but potentially changeable, reaction of a system attracted to something else. If we can change the attractors or tap into existing ones that are better, the system may do the rest of the work of change on its own. The challenge for managers is to then look for the subtle attractors that may not always be obvious.

Using the CAS framework, Plsek (2001) suggests it is more helpful to think like a farmer than an engineer. Engineers design every detail of a system, which is possible because the parts are mechanical and predictable. Farmers know they can do only so much. Farmers use knowledge and past experience to create conditions under which a good crop is possible. The outcome, an emergent property of the natural system, cannot be predicted in detail. This concept will be applied later to the development of continuous readiness programs.

Consistent with this understanding of organizations as complex adaptive systems, Zimmerman et al. (2001) propose practical principles of management for the real world that are new ways of thinking about our roles as quality leaders in organizations. These principles are outlined briefly in **Figure 3-1** and are later applied to the process of creating continuous readiness.

B. Changing Organizational Culture to One of Readiness

Culture is a system of beliefs and actions that characterize a particular group (O'Toole, 1996). An organization's culture is the complex interrelated whole of standardized, institutionalized, habitual behavior that characterizes that organization. Culture also refers to norms of behavior and shared values among a group of people (Kotter, 1996). *Norms of behavior* are common or pervasive ways of acting that are found in a group. They persist because group members tend to behave in ways that teach these practices to new members, rewarding those who fit in and penalizing those who do not. *Shared values* are important concerns and goals shared by most of the people in a group; they tend to shape group behavior

Figure 3-1. Management Principles for Complex Adaptive Systems (CAS)

Complexity lens	View systems through the lens of complexity in addition to using traditional metaphors such as a machine or a military organization. This can be stress-reducing, as many of the changes in healthcare cannot be predicted in CAS. Learning to be flexible and adaptable is the only sustainable leadership strategy.
Good-enough vision	Build a good-enough vision and provide minimum specifications rather than trying to plan out every little detail. By the time detailed plans are complete, the assumptions and inputs must be changed almost immediately. Complexity science suggests that people should be better off with minimum specifications and a general sense of direction, thus allowing appropriate autonomy for individuals to self-organize and adapt as time goes by.
Clockware/ swarmware	Balance data and intuition, planning and acting, safety and risk, giving due significance to each. Describe the absolute boundaries and let the people become active in trying whatever they think might work.
"Tune to the edge"	Tune the organization to the edge by fostering the right degree of information flow, diversity and difference, connections inside and outside the organization, power differential and anxiety; instead of controlling information, forcing agreement, dealing separately with contentious groups, working systematically down all the layers of the hierarchy in sequence, and seeking comfort.
Paradox	Uncover and work with paradox and tension rather than shying away from them as if they were unnatural. Creativity and innovation have the best chance to emerge precisely at the point of greatest tension and seemingly irreconcilable differences.
Multiple actions	Go for multiple actions at the fringes, let direction arise rather than believing that there must be certainty before anything proceeds. Allow the flexibility of multiple approaches.
Shadow system	Listen to the "shadow system," realizing that informal relationships, gossip, rumor, and hallway conversations contribute significantly to agents' mental models and subsequent actions. This shadow system, rather than the formal hierarchy, has diversity of thought and approach. This often is the place where creativity resides in an organization.
Chunking	Grow complex systems by allowing them to emerge out of the links among simple systems that work well and are capable of operating independently. A good approach to building complex systems is to start small, experiment to get pieces (chunks) that work, and then link the pieces together.
Competition/ cooperation	Mix cooperation and competition. Nature competes and nature cooperates; these dynamics are not mutually exclusive.

Source: Zimmerman et al., 2001.

and often persist over time even when group membership changes. Culture is important because it can powerfully influence human behavior, because it can be difficult to change, and because its "invisibility" makes it hard to address directly.

General, shared values, which are less apparent but more deeply ingrained in the culture, are more difficult to change than norms of behavior. Culture changes only after people's actions have been successfully altered, after the new behavior produces some group benefit for a period of time, and after people see the connection between the new actions and the performance improvement.

People generally are unaware of their organizational culture until it is challenged, until they experience a new culture, or until it is made overt and explicit through a framework or model (Cameron & Quinn, 1999). Inside an organization, subunits such as functional departments, hierarchical levels, or even teams also may reflect their own unique cultures. Difficulties in coordinating and integrating processes or organizational activities often are a result of culture clashes among different subunits. Cultural differences can fragment an organization and make high levels of effectiveness impossible to achieve.

Modifying organizational culture is a key to the successful implementation of major improvement strategies, as well as adaptation to the increasing turbulent environment faced by modern organizations (Cameron & Quinn, 1999). The failure rate of most planned organizational change initiatives is dramatic. Several studies reported that the most frequently cited reason given for failure was a neglect of the organization's culture (failure to change the organization's culture doomed the other kinds of organizational changes that were initiated; Cameron, 1995; Cameron & Ettington, 1988). Organizational culture has a powerful effect on the performance and long-term effectiveness of organizations. In addition to organization-level effects, the impact of organizational culture on individuals (employee morale, commitment, productivity, health, and well-being) is well-documented (Cameron, Freeman, & Mishra, 1991; Kozlowski, Chao, Smith, & Hedlund, 1993).

Cultural change is intimately tied to individual change. To change culture is to change oneself, not changing "it" or "them" (O'Toole, 1996). Unless managers are willing to commit to personal change, the organization's culture will remain recalcitrant (Cameron & Quinn, 1999). Many efforts fail because the organization's fundamental culture—the values, the ways of thinking, the managerial styles, the paradigms, and approaches to problem solving—remains the same. This dependence of organizational improvement on culture change is due to the fact that when the values, orientations, definitions, and goals stay constant, even when procedures and strategies are altered, organizations return quickly to the status quo. The same is true for individuals. Without an alteration of the fundamental goals, values, and expectations of organizations or individuals, change remains superficial and short-term in duration.

Altering the culture of a corporation is slow, hard work (O'Toole, 1996). Leaders need the patience to involve the entire organization in the process of change and need time to do it. Daniels and Mathers (1997) suggest that significant results can be experienced in 6 to 9 months, but complete transformations usually take at least 2 or 3 years. Implementing a culture of continuous readiness cannot be done overnight, and quality leaders must be patient and persistent to see the transformation through.

C. Leading Readiness Change

To effect true change, one must become a leader of leaders, one who inspires others to lead the transformation (O'Toole, 1996). Such leadership is difficult because there is no formula and one must be willing, for starters, to change oneself.

While management is a set of processes that can keep a complex system of people and technology running smoothly, leadership defines what the future should look like, aligns people with that vision, and inspires them to make it happen despite the obstacles (Kotter, 1996). This distinction is crucial, as successful transformation is 70%–90% leadership and only 10%–30% management. An emphasis on management rather than leadership often has been institutionalized in corporate cultures that discourage employees from learning how to lead. Managing change is important because without competent management, the transformation process can become out of control. But for most organizations, the much bigger challenge is leading change. Leadership often begins with just one or two people, but that number needs to grow over time. Modern organizations are far too complex to be transformed by a single "larger-than-life" individual. Many people need to help with the leadership task by assisting with the leadership agenda in their own spheres of activity.

O'Toole (1996) shares the analyses of successful leaders over time. He identified the following themes from studying many successful leaders from a variety of industries: enabling others to lead by sharing information; fostering a sense of community; and creating a consistent system of rewards, structure, process, and communication. They were committed to the principle of opportunity, giving all followers the chance to make a contribution to the organization. The values-based leadership they all practiced was based on an inspiring vision. Each was dedicated to institutionalizing continuous change, renewal, innovation, and learning. The bottom line in what they did was to adhere to the moral principle of respect for people. In all the examples cited, the leaders used different methods to create change—there was no single formula. Institutionalized change processes took as long as 10 years to show clear results. All of the changes, however, entailed one form or another of decentralization of decision making, monitoring of stakeholder needs, challenging of assumptions, and providing appropriate rewards and incentives for all of these activities. In each case, the process began with a clear, long-term, top-management commitment to the hard work of altering corporate culture, beginning with themselves.

Kotter (1996) provides an eight-stage process of creating major change (**Figure 3-2**), which addresses errors common to organizational change efforts. Common errors cited include the following:

- allowing too much complacency
- failing to create a sufficiently powerful guiding coalition
- underestimating the power of vision
- undercommunicating the vision
- permitting obstacles to block the new vision
- failing to create short-term wins
- declaring victory too soon
- neglecting to anchor changes firmly in the corporate culture.

The first four steps in the process help "defrost" a hardened status quo; the next three phases introduce many new practices; and the last stage grounds the changes in the corporate culture and helps make them stick. Successful change goes through all eight stages, usually in sequence although it is normal to go through multiple

Figure 3-2. Eight-Stage Process of Creating Major Change

1 **Establishing a sense of urgency:** Examining the market and competitive realities; identifying and discussing crises, potential crises, or major opportunities.

2 **Creating the guiding coalition:** Putting together a group with enough power to lead the change (key characteristics are position power, expertise, credibility, and leadership); getting the group to work together like a team to make change happen (find the right people, create trust, and develop a common goal).

3 **Developing a vision and strategy:** Creating a vision to help direct the change effort and developing strategies to achieve that vision. Vision clarifies the general direction for change; it motivates people to take action in the right direction, and it helps coordinate the actions of different people in an efficient way. An effective vision is imaginable, desirable, feasible, focused, flexible, and communicable.

4 **Communicating the change vision:** Using every vehicle possible to constantly communicate the new vision and strategies; having the guiding coalition role-model the behavior expected of employees. Effective communication of the vision requires simplicity (no jargon), a verbal picture or metaphor, multiple forums to spread the word, repetition, leadership by example, explanation of apparent inconsistencies, and two-way communication.

5 **Empowering broad-based action:** Getting rid of obstacles; changing systems or structures that undermine the change vision; encouraging risk-taking and nontraditional ideas, activities, and actions. Employees are an enormous source of power to improve organizational performance. Empowering people to effect change requires leadership to communicate a sensible vision to employees, make structures compatible with the vision, provide the training employees need, align information and personnel systems to the vision, and confront supervisors who undercut needed change.

6 **Generating short-term wins:** Planning for visible improvements in performance, or "wins"; creating those wins; visibly recognizing and rewarding people who made the wins possible. A good short-term win is visible to large numbers of people, is unambiguous, and is clearly related to the change effort. Short-term performance improvements help transformations in the following ways: provide evidence that sacrifices are worth it, reward change agents with a "pat on the back," help fine-tune vision and strategies, undermine cynics and self-serving resisters, keep bosses on board, and build momentum.

7 **Consolidating gains and producing more change:** Using increased credibility to change all systems, structures, and policies that don't fit together and don't fit the transformation vision; hiring, promoting, and developing people who can implement the change vision; reinvigorating the process with new projects, themes, and change agents. Changing anything of significance in highly interdependent systems often means changing nearly everything—transformation can become a huge exercise that takes place over years, not months. Outstanding leaders are willing to think long-term—they are willing to stay the course to accomplish objectives that are important. Without sufficient leadership, change stalls.

8 **Anchoring new approaches in the culture:** Creating better performance through customer- and productivity-oriented behavior, more and better leadership, and more effective management; articulating the connections between new behaviors and organizational success; developing means to ensure leadership development and succession. When new practices are not compatible with the relevant cultures, they will always be subject to regression. Anchoring changes comes last in the transformation, not first; it depends on results and requires a lot of discussion; it may involve turnover; and leadership succession decisions are crucial.

Source: Kotter, 1996.

phases at once. Most major change initiatives are made up of a number of smaller projects, with each going through the multistep process. So at any one time, people might be halfway through the overall effort, finished with a few smaller pieces, and just beginning other projects. Thus, with multiple steps and multiple projects, the end result is often complex, dynamic, and messy rather than a simple linear analytical process (in other words, a complex adaptive system).

D. Creating Continuous Readiness in Complex Organizations

Application of these frameworks for leading change within complex organizations can be useful for healthcare quality professionals leading an organization toward a culture of continuous readiness. By using Kotter's (1996) eight-stage change process and applying Zimmerman and colleagues' (2001) management principles for complex organizations, the process for creating a corporate culture of continuous readiness was developed. **Figure 3-3** outlines eight steps in a process to guide the creation of this culture, which is the foundation of a successful continuous readiness program.

IV. Continuous Readiness Programs

For many healthcare quality professionals, previous survey preparations used a just-in-time model that required ramp-up activities in the months prior to the survey to ensure success. Most organizations required tremendous additional resources in order to be successful, such as extra time, energy, and people; as well as extra meetings for policy revision approvals and education on standards, roles, and survey process. The organizations approached training for staff using just-in-time planning to ensure that education wasn't premature (staff might forget before the survey). Most organizations experienced tremendous relief when surveys were over and many committed to a vision that the next 2- or 3-year cycle would be different, yet the organization's culture was one in which a 2- or 3-year hiatus was expected until the next ramp-up. Healthcare quality professionals may have found it difficult to get leadership's attention for identified compliance issues after a survey, especially in those organizations that did well during the previous survey. These same organizations also may experience unplanned surveys or regulatory visits that don't go as well and, even with the best of intentions, a crisis management cycle inevitably begins, which requires additional resources to regain compliance.

The goal of continuous readiness programs is to break crisis management cycles and just-in-time cultures to provide continuous safe quality patient care and sustained compliance with evidence-based practices, professional standards, and regulations. As noted earlier in discussion of the CAS framework, Plsek (2001) suggests it is more helpful to think like a farmer than an engineer. Engineers design every detail of a system, which is possible because the parts are mechanical and predictable. Farmers know they can only do so much and use knowledge and past experience to create conditions under which a good crop is possible. Application in this case is for a good survey and continuous compliance demonstration. Key components of successful readiness programs include leadership commitment, manager accountability, routine self-assessment, corrective action plan development and monitoring, new standard or regulation oversight, staff education, staff recognition, survey preparation processes, and unannounced visit or survey plans.

Figure 3-3. Eight-Stage Process of Creating Continuous Readiness in Complex Organizations

1 **Establishing a sense of urgency**
- Highlight competitive realities that drive the need for high-quality, safe patient care.
- Conduct cost analyses for resources invested in previous crisis management or survey preparations.
- Examine employee morale and turnover (at all levels in the organization) that result from the current culture of crisis management.
- Engage senior leaders in discussion of current and potential crises and major opportunities to improve readiness and compliance.
- Determine if top management or senior leadership has the long-term commitment to the hard work of altering the organization's culture.
- Determine if senior leaders are willing to change their own behaviors.
- Identify shared values related to a culture of readiness, and make them explicit to build on the organization's existing culture.

2 **Creating the guiding coalition**
- Enlist individuals with enough power and leadership skill to lead the change. Balance the group with individuals with positions of power, expertise, credibility, and leadership.
- Create trust within the group and a common goal.
- Remember to balance data and intuition, planning and acting, safety and risk.
- Identify key stakeholders for a culture of readiness and the attractors for each stakeholder group.
- Define the absolute boundaries to let people become active in trying whatever they think might work.
- Uncover and work with paradox and tension.
- "Tune to the edge" by fostering the right degree of information flow, diversity and difference, connections inside/outside the organization, power differential, and anxiety; instead of controlling information, forcing agreement, dealing separately with contentious groups, working systematically down all the layers of the hierarchy in sequence.

3 **Developing a vision and strategy**
- Create a continuous readiness vision, such as "A company/corporate attitude and value of continuous compliance."
- Create a continuous readiness mission, such as "An uninterrupted state of being mentally prepared and immediately (physically) ready to demonstrate compliance."
- Develop a mental picture of what readiness would look like in the organization (and what it would not look like), emphasizing shared values.
- Define long-term and short-term goals to achieve readiness.
- Develop strategies to achieve the vision within the organization and culture.
- Develop a plan to grow leaders.
- Remain focused on attractors for key stakeholders to use the organization's natural energy.
- Identify past practices that have been barriers or obstacles to the vision.
- Identify behaviors that support the vision, which will be important for managers and leaders to role-model.
- Remember to view systems through the "complexity" lens—be flexible and adaptable.

4 **Communicating the change vision**
- Determine every vehicle possible to constantly communicate the vision and strategies.
- Describe what readiness will look like in the organization.
- Role-model behaviors expected of employees.
- Engage in two-way communication with staff at all levels.
- Listen to the shadow system for diversity of thought, approach, and creativity.
- Listen to key stakeholders and their evolving needs.
- Describe stories that highlight behaviors that support the vision.

continued

Figure 3-3. Eight-Stage Process of Creating Continuous Readiness in Complex Organizations *(continued)*

5 **Empowering broad-based action**

- Implement the strategy and plans for growing leaders.
- Remove obstacles.
- Change systems or structures that undermine the vision.
- Encourage risk-taking and nontraditional ideas, activities, and actions.
- Provide employee training.
- Confront supervisors who undermine the needed changes.
- Use "good-enough" vision and provide minimum specifications rather than planning every detail.
- Allow autonomy.
- Provide opportunity to allow others a chance to make a contribution.
- Teach employees how to lead in their spheres of activities.
- "Tune to the edge" by fostering the right degree of information flow, diversity and difference, connections inside/outside the organization, power differential, and anxiety; instead of controlling information, forcing agreement, dealing separately with contentious groups, working systematically down all the layers of the hierarchy in sequence.
- Go for multiple actions at the fringes; let direction arise rather than believing that there must be certainty before anything proceeds.
- Implement rapid and small tests of change in processes.
- Allow the flexibility of multiple approaches.
- Grow complex systems by allowing them to emerge out of the links among simple systems that work well and are capable of operating independently.
- Mix cooperation and competition.

6 **Generating short-term wins**

- Plan for visible improvements in performance—often the small tests of change.
- Create wins.
- Describe stories of actions or changes that support the vision with which staff can identify.
- Visibly recognize and reward people who made wins possible.
- Go for multiple actions at the fringes; let direction arise rather than believing that there must be certainty before anything proceeds.
- Allow the flexibility of multiple approaches.
- Grow complex systems by allowing them to emerge out of the links among simple systems that work well and are capable of operating independently.
- Mix cooperation and competition.

7 **Consolidating gains and producing more change**

- Change all systems, structures, and policies that don't fit the transformation.
- Hire, promote, and develop people who can implement the vision.
- Reinvigorate the process with new projects and change agents.
- Stay the course; the process takes time.
- Remember to view systems through the complexity lens—be flexible and adaptable.
- Uncover and work with paradox and tension.
- Describe stories of actions or changes that support the vision with which staff can identify.
- Visibly recognize and reward people who made wins possible.

8 **Anchoring new approaches in the culture**

- Articulate the connections between new behaviors and organizational success.
- Create better performance.
- Describe stories of actions or changes that support the vision with which staff can identify.
- Visibly recognize and reward people who made wins possible.
- Develop means to ensure leadership development and succession.
- Grow complex systems by allowing them to emerge out of the links among simple systems that work well and are capable of operating independently.

A. Leadership Commitment

Leadership commitment to continuous readiness must be in place for programs to be successful. Leaders must be willing to change their organization's culture to one of readiness, which requires the leaders to commit to personal change and create an environment where the values, ways of thinking, managerial styles, paradigms, and approaches to problem solving support a culture of readiness. Leaders must be patient and persistent to see this transformation through by defining what readiness looks like within their organization, aligning staff with that vision, and inspiring staff to make it happen despite obstacles that will surface. Figure 3-3, the eight-stage process of creating continuous readiness in complex organizations, provides a guide for this work.

To commit, leaders must understand the business case for compliance and understand the costs of noncompliance. Costs may be known from previous ramp-up activities or noncompliance situations, or there may be potential costs from adverse media attention and loss of patients or business. With the expanding culture of public reporting of quality and performance measures, organizations are subject to scrutiny from a variety of perspectives once media attention is drawn to them. The business case for continuous readiness also includes the impact on staff of ramp-up activities and crisis compliance management. Staff and managers can experience frustration and burnout with crisis compliance management and seek employment elsewhere, thus depleting organizations of experienced employees (those who possess crucial institutional memory).

Leaders must include continuous readiness within organizational strategic priorities in order to change the culture. It must be part of the operational budgeting process, part of key leadership activities, and a key topic that leaders inquire about in routine discussions with staff and managers. Leaders also must be willing to hold managers accountable for readiness responsibilities.

B. Manager Accountability

Managers play a key role in continuous readiness activities. Compliance is evaluated by what happens to patients at the point of care delivery. Policies and procedures can provide the guidance and structure for those providing or supporting care delivery, but actual practice and policies must be aligned to achieve compliance.

Healthcare quality professionals in leadership roles cannot be the lone voices requiring compliance in complex organizations. The management team provides operational oversight within an organization and is the key to ensuring continuous compliance within their areas of accountability. Healthcare quality professionals must provide the program structure and education to help managers understand their accountabilities and be successful. New managers have steep learning curves to understand not only their departmental operations but also functional interrelatedness and regulatory and accreditation standards. As they learn to juggle operations, fiscal accountabilities, staffing, and patient relations, they also must incorporate compliance into their busy days. Unfortunately, it may be easier to allocate time to the faces and duties of the given day, rather than to proactive readiness accountabilities. Thus, the culture of the organization and the strategic priority placed on readiness will be determining factors in the success of readiness programs.

C. Routine Self-assessment

Routine self-assessment is a cornerstone of continuous readiness programs. The ability to evaluate compliance of key regulatory and accreditation standards is a critical step in the process. In the just-in-time scenario discussed earlier, compliance is not sustained, but fluctuates in response to known survey cycles. Compliance improves immediately before a survey and gradually declines after each survey. The goal of continuous readiness programs is to sustain compliance. To do this, an organization must evaluate its compliance state periodically. Two common assessment models are discussed below.

1. Annual Assessment

With an annual assessment model, organizations plan for a thorough assessment once per calendar year, often at the beginning of a fiscal year. Resources are dedicated for the review, whether conducted internally or by an external consultant, as time is required for content experts to conduct actual reviews and document their findings. In this model, an assessment is completed and presented to leadership and quality oversight committees and often to an organization's board of directors/trustees. Ideally, this report is in the format of a gap analysis related to specific standards, with findings and recommendations written in a manner that facilitates corrective action planning. Once the findings are presented, corrective action plans must be developed and monitored on an ongoing basis. Many organizations find that monthly or bimonthly status reports on corrective actions provide the oversight necessary to ensure course correction to achieve compliance. Using quarterly status reports runs the risk that the organization will not be aware of slippage. The advantage of an annual assessment is that the assessment is planned, resourced, and completed in a relatively short period of time allowing for action plan development, implementation, and monitoring throughout the remainder of the year. This model lends itself to assistance from resources such as internal corporate or external consultants who facilitate the rapid completion of the assessment. A disadvantage of this model is that it requires dedicated resources to complete the assessment within a defined short period of time, as opposed to integration into other organizational activities or duties.

2. Ongoing Assessment

With an ongoing assessment model, organizations plan for a thorough assessment over the calendar year, often dividing the workload over the entire year with monthly activities scheduled. Resources may not be dedicated for the review; rather, responsibility may be an additional duty assigned to existing staff (one or many), and time is taken from other accountabilities to complete tasks within the scheduled timeline. Documentation of findings for leadership action may be done centrally by one person or department or by each person completing an assessment segment using a reporting template. In this model, as the assessment components are completed, they should be presented to leadership and quality oversight committees rather than at completion of the assessment cycle. Presentation to the organization's board of directors/trustees can be periodic or at the end of the assessment cycle and can be a summary of the assessment components rather than an individual completed report. This report is most useful when in the format of a gap analysis related to specific standards, with findings and recommendations written in a manner that facilitates rapid corrective action planning. Once the findings are presented, corrective action plans must be developed and monitored on an ongoing basis. Monitoring schedules in this model are more complex, as they must incorporate scheduled assessments to be completed as well as follow-up activities on those that have been completed. Many organizations find that monthly or twice-monthly status reports on assessment components and corrective actions provide the oversight necessary to ensure course correction to achieve compliance. Quarterly status reports are not recommended with this model because there is a high risk that the organization will not be aware of slippage. The advantage of an ongoing assessment is that the assessment can be integrated into ongoing operational activities and reported over an ongoing (but defined) period of time, allowing for action plan development, implementation, and monitoring throughout the year. This model lends itself to integration into existing operations. A disadvantage of this model is that it requires focused project management to ensure completion of the entire assessment and to ensure monitoring and oversight of required corrective actions. There is a risk of not completing the entire assessment. It also may be difficult for the organization to have a "snapshot" of compliance to understand performance.

Accrediting agencies often have tools available to help organizations manage self-assessment activities. Easily accessible and easy-to-use checklists may be available on agency Intranet sites. Additional paper-based or computer-based project management programs designed specifically for the identified accreditation program also may be purchased from most agencies. External consulting organizations also will provide educational programs or tools when their services are retained for preparation activities.

D. Corrective Action Plans

Corrective action plans, *plans of corrections*, *improvement plans*, and *action plans* are terms used to describe documents that organize improvements needed for organizations to be in full compliance with standards or regulations. These plans often are written in response to a survey, inspection, or gap analyses from assessments that define observations as well as recommendations for actions to achieve compliance for a given standard. Documents also may be created proactively at the discretion of leadership to address upcoming changes in standards or regulations. Plans often are coordinated by a central person or department (often the quality and performance improvement department), but may receive input from many different departments or staff.

These documents are commonly formatted into a table or a grid. Typical columns in the table are for the topic or standard, issue/finding/observation of the current state of compliance, planned actions, timeline for completion, and the name of the person accountable for the action. It is increasingly common for complex documents to also include a column for the oversight body or committee and a schedule for status reports. This approach is useful for large projects where it becomes difficult to manage the status of each topic. Rows in the table or grid address individual improvement areas or topics. Tables are useful documents to assist with project management as they may be sorted by columns to organize the work by topic, by deadline, or by the person responsible for completing the task.

Development of an appropriate and feasible action plan is only the beginning of an effective continuous readiness program. The most difficult part of the program is oversight of action plans to ensure that they are fully implemented, evaluated, and revised as necessary until full compliance is achieved and sustained. Leadership prioritization and support and a culture of readiness are factors that will influence success. Healthcare quality professionals can facilitate explicit communication related to accountability expectations and timelines for completion and oversight reporting. They also can ensure tracking systems for required status reports to be prepared for oversight bodies. Healthcare quality professionals must also take responsibility when evaluations provide evidence that actions are not successful and further measures may be required. Leadership cannot facilitate the removal of obstacles and barriers of which they are not aware.

E. New Standard Oversight

One of the most important components of a continuous readiness program is a defined process to ensure that the organization is aware of changes in standards or regulations. Changes may be in the form of additions, deletions, or enhancements to scoring guidelines. Most regulatory or accreditation agencies have defined processes for changes; these usually involve notification to the affected organizations and a period of time where comments or feedback on proposed changes are accepted prior to their publication. Healthcare quality professionals should check with the agencies and organizations that survey their facilities to understand

- the relative frequency with which changes are made
- the process for assimilating "public" feedback and comments from affected organizations
- the notification process to the affected organizations, including the medium (e-mail, paper letter, Web site announcements) and whom in the organization communications should be directed to (e.g., the Chief Executive Officer).

Once changes are identified, internal oversight committees will need to be made aware and staff education will be required. It is helpful to create a notification list of individuals within the organization who should receive communications related to standards. These communications are most effective when they are put into context for the recipient. For example, the communication should include a description of the change, the agency making the change, actions required on the part of the recipient, risk assessment of the change, and deadlines associated with required actions.

F. Staff Education

Continuous readiness programs require solid staff education programs with participation from all levels and all areas within an organization. Healthcare quality professionals must develop an effective and efficient education plan that targets defined levels within the organization:

- senior leaders must receive information to prioritize resources for readiness and to speak to key leadership standards when surveyors visit their facilities
- front-line staff must receive information to comply with standards and regulations related to direct care delivery
- the management team must have information related to care delivery, structure or process standards, as well as standard changes and associated implications.

Healthcare quality professionals also must develop an effective education plan that targets defined departments within an organization. For example, key messages for large departments such as nursing may be different from key messages for smaller ancillary departments; or key messages for surgical departments may be different from those for maternity units. If programs are not designed specifically for an intended audience, participants may believe that the majority of the material applies to another department or may be unable to apply the message to their own department. Organizations may have education departments that can help design these programs and provide the structure for delivery.

In previous models of survey preparation, the majority of education was planned as just-in-time training—not too far in advance of a survey, so as not to run the risk of staff or leaders forgetting the information prior to survey, and not too close in time to the actual survey, when staff and leaders become overwhelmed with information. Pocket guides or booklets have been popular vehicles for this type of education, as well as quick reference attachments to name badges. Although there is still a place for just-in-time education before announced surveys, the focus of this training in a continuous readiness program should be on what staff and leaders can expect to take place during an actual survey. For example, just-in-time education may be effective to inform staff what the survey agenda will look like, types and numbers of surveyors or inspectors to expect, planned interview sessions (who will participate and anticipated topics), and documents that might be required during the survey process.

Successful continuous readiness programs are an outcome of staff having been creative in developing vehicles for education to reach staff and leaders, and effec-tively imparting key messages and reinforcing them across the organization. Classroom training sessions continue to be used in most organizations; these programs require conference room space to allow large numbers of participants, as well as flexible program scheduling to allow participants with various shift and work schedules to participate. Newsletters also have been used successfully to reach staff on two or three different shifts and with 7-day operations (paper newsletters suit the culture of many organizations, while others find them onerous to create and publish regularly, and the printing costs to be prohibitive). Storyboards or poster boards placed in key locations throughout the facility can efficiently educate staff and patients or customers alike, and can be created inexpensively using desktop publishing programs such as Microsoft PowerPoint®. Large organizations may have teleconferencing capability to broadcast educational programs throughout an organization's multiple campuses; these also can be taped and viewed after the initial broadcast for ongoing training purposes. Teleconferencing technology has improved to allow moderators to manage multiple telephone lines and still produce effective audio conferences with large numbers of participants. Many organizations have transitioned to Intranet or Internet training programs that can be viewed directly from a computer station and heard through the computer or associated telephone lines. Internet or computer-based learning programs also are an effective tool.

Healthcare quality professionals have also been creative in developing effective ongoing programs when workforces are constantly changing. One tool for development of ongoing programs and flexible program scheduling has been the use of train-the-trainer educational sessions. This option allows a program to be developed and taught to those who will in turn teach the program to others. For example, healthcare quality professionals might sponsor a program for all managers, who in turn will be responsible for teaching the program to their individual unit staff. This is an effective method to reach large numbers of staff on varying shifts and schedules, but it depends on the commitment of each manager to follow through. Self-study modules, whether paper-based, computer-based, or video-based, also are efficient means to deliver standardized, ongoing education.

Creating fun educational programs is an essential part of successful continuous readiness programs. Staff members appreciate an opportunity to make learning fun, and developing incentives through competitions can help to generate enthusiasm for the program. Television game shows with "survival" tactics or a question-answer format have served as models for programs; board games and crossword puzzles also have been used successfully. Healthcare quality professionals can use this as an opportunity to exercise their creativity.

Education calendars should be planned in advance as a cohesive program rather than as a series of seemingly unrelated topics. Education programs can be designed around survey cycles over 2 or 3 years. The following is an example of an education program organized around a survey cycle.

1. Year One (Pre-survey)

The focus of this year could be to keep staff and leadership apprised of key standards and regulations and any anticipated changes, and the associated agencies that survey the organization. Programs planned throughout the year could highlight functions or clusters of topics for defined audiences. For example, a series might be planned for managers and leaders, highlighting accountabilities that cross department boundaries, such as

- sentinel event policies
- patient safety goals
- patient rights and responsibilities topics
- medication management
- infection control practices
- employee safety programs
- environment of care management
- human resource expectations
- performance improvement programs
- unannounced survey procedures.

Another series might be planned for medical staff, highlighting

- key topics from the bylaws
- key standards or regulations that relate specifically to the medical staff functions (e.g., peer review privileging, sedation practices, patient safety goals, patient rights or privacy rules)
- quality initiatives tied to outcome measures for clinical diagnostic groups
- public reporting agendas related to outcome measures and the associated initiatives to improve them.

A series might also be planned for front-line staff, taught by managers and leaders who have participated in train-the-trainer programs, highlighting topics such as

- national and regional patient safety goals
- patient rights and responsibilities topics
- medication management
- infection control practices
- employee safety programs
- environment of care management
- performance improvement programs (highlighting visible improvements in performance).

A series of programs to build skills related to regulatory, accreditation, or quality improvement should also be considered. Examples of skill-building programs might be topics related to

- basic business knowledge to highlight competitive realities that drive the need for high-quality, safe patient care

- quality improvement models
- improvement team facilitation
- committee management (facilitation, chairmanship, committee support and organization, minutes)
- overview of regulatory and accrediting organizations or agencies
- change management (including programs that teach employees to lead within their spheres of activities).

2. Year Two (Survey Year)

The focus of this year could be to prepare staff and leadership for anticipated survey activities. Kick-off educational programs might incorporate basic information around the planned survey to educate staff about the purpose of the survey, the value of the survey to the organization, expected timelines for the survey (dates), and expectations of staff, managers, and physicians during the survey process. Survey etiquette should be included as a topic, including measures of appropriate behavior during the actual survey and pointers on how to interact with surveyors.

Mid-year programs might emphasize "hot topics" or key standards or regulations that will be a focus during the survey, with information about how the organization complies, and information about performance improvement initiatives related to the key topics. There also should be a focus on programs that the organization is proud of and success stories from the field. All staff should be aware of the organization's good work and be able to express their pride in the organization during the survey.

End-of-the-year programs might focus on practice sessions for known interviews or survey sessions to help staff feel comfortable while participating in the actual survey. Follow-up programs might focus on the survey results, opportunities identified for improvement, and anticipated action plans associated with these findings.

3. Year Three (Post-survey Year)

The focus of this year could be very similar to the focus of the first year, with the addition of programs that highlight survey results and next steps associated with opportunities identified for improvement, as well as new programs associated with these opportunities or findings.

G. Staff Recognition

Staff recognition and rewards for participation in continuous readiness programs have been cited as success factors for many programs. Staff members experience an ever-increasing list of tasks they must accomplish and documentation they must complete, while trying to meet organizational expectations for efficiency and customer service. Participation in proactive readiness or crisis-prevention activities may not appear to be a top priority unless there is a culture of readiness. Some steps in achieving this culture are to discuss actions or changes that support the vision, and to recognize and reward people who made short-terms wins possible. Recognition can be simple and still be effective. Leadership acknowledgment through personal words of thanks, notes of appreciation, or public acknowledgment in committees or meetings are all effective means of recognition. Timely recognition, even if simple, may be more effective than waiting for formal recognition forums that are few and far between and may not be well-attended. Simple rewards can still be effective. Small treats such as candy, or trinkets such as pens or pins, or coupons for coffee or lunch, are appreciated by staff on all shifts and are most effective if given at the time of participation. Leadership rounds on the clinical units are also an effective way to acknowledge staff members and to solicit their input and feedback on further opportunities to support and improve the continuous readiness programs.

H. Survey Preparation Processes

Healthcare quality professionals develop and manage the survey preparation process for the organization; serve as internal consultants for the organization; and coordinate survey preparation with the assistance of all leaders, managers, and staff. The coordination required to achieve favorable accreditation status or successful regulatory licensing or certifications must be delegated to those individuals with the most knowledge about evidence-based care, healthcare quality, regulations, and standards interpretation and implementation. Important tasks for organizations to complete for survey preparation are generally outlined in accreditation manuals.

1. Survey Initiation

The first step in survey preparation is to initiate the application for a survey; each agency has a unique process for accomplishing its survey. Expect an application process for a new licensing survey or an initial accreditation survey, as well as a reapplication process for continuing or renewing licensing or accreditation. Agencies often have application information readily available in publications or on Internet sites that help guide facilities through an often-tedious process. Reviewing applications far in advance may be helpful to fully understand the data needed to describe the services included in the survey. Survey fees may be required during the application process, or they may be billed after the survey is completed. Many applications can now be completed electronically through the Internet and secure Web sites, and some agencies such as the Joint Commission or NCQA now require electronic application processes. Inquire with the agency in advance as to the options that are available for application submission, deadlines for submission, anticipated fees, and required signatures.

After the application has been submitted, the agencies initiate the survey planning process from their perspective. The actual survey may begin prior to on-site survey activities through "desktop review"—the submission of materials electronically or the mailing of documents for review by the survey team in advance of arrival. Understanding submission requirements is critical to a successful survey; it ensures that documents focus on the surveying agency's specific criteria. Existing documents may lack the focus required for submission within defined page limits or within form boundaries. In addition, performance data, complaint data, news articles, financial statements, and other publicly available data may be gathered by the agency to help prioritize areas of focus during the on-site survey process. Expect requests for additional information or clarifying information prior to the on-site survey.

2. Survey Coordination

The survey coordinator facilitates collaboration among the departments and services in demonstrating compliance with the standards. The best way to prepare for a survey is through the formation of a multidisciplinary accreditation team. The team's composition will vary depending on the type of provider (e.g., hospital, managed care organization, long-term-care facility, home healthcare agency, or ambulatory care center). At a minimum, the team should consist of the healthcare quality professional and representatives from administration, nursing, key ancillary departments, medical staff, and the governing board. In the hospital setting, other members might include the safety officer, risk manager, and director of health information management/medical records. In a managed care organization, additional members might include customer relations, physician relations/medical staff coordinator, information systems/data processing, and the benefits administrator. The increasing role and accountability of the medical staff in performance improvement and accreditation make it essential that they receive enough lead time to clear their schedules. Most accrediting organizations have generic survey schedules that are available to the organization approximately 4 months prior to the date of the survey.

The frequency with which the accreditation team meets will vary depending on the outcome of ongoing self-assessments and available resources to complete identified tasks. The team can help to ensure a smooth survey with careful planning. If the team has performed its duties in a continuous fashion and the organization has created a culture of readiness, the last-minute rush and accompanying stress will be lessened. The team's attention can then be focused in the last few weeks on the details of the actual survey, such as conducting just-in-time training. A number of publications with suggested checklists to assist with survey preparation are available. Each of the accrediting agencies as well as independent consulting/educational companies provide educational programs on survey preparation. The most important element, however, is a coordinated, ongoing effort to meet the standards; this will provide the best results. The activities listed below are examples of duties that multidisciplinary accreditation teams and the survey coordinator can oversee for scheduled surveys.

- Complete survey applications by posted deadlines, allowing time to obtain required signatures of senior leaders.
- Update lists of phone numbers and create e-mail distribution lists, phone distribution lists, and pager distribution lists to facilitate rapid communication during the survey. Develop organizational charts that can be attached to the phone lists to have the correct title available. Set up a distribution for digital messaging if the facility has text pager or phone systems.
- Determine staffing plans for survey dates. Clarify vacation expectations of key staff and leaders based on known survey dates. Review physician staffing plans for the weeks preceding and during the survey to ensure medical staff participation. Review staffing plans with leadership for the weeks preceding and during the survey. Pull operating room schedules for the days prior to and during the survey to identify the staff who will be on duty during the survey, and check the credentials of all identified personnel.
- Check quality data available to the surveyors in advance. Be sure leaders are aware of these data and how the organization performs, and are able to speak about improvement initiatives related to these data.
- Review previous survey findings and DHS or CMS reports and the respective corrective action plans to evaluate that the gains were held.
- Ensure that the most current licenses, certificates, patient rights posters, Emergency Medical Treatment and Active Labor Act (EMTALA) signs, and other materials are posted.
- Identify the location of key documents that may be required during the survey.
- Review policies and procedures to ensure all are current, including departmental documents.

- Conduct chart reviews of open records to ensure compliant records. Concurrent chart review should be occurring on a consistent basis. If a record has been thinned, ensure that the appropriate information is included in the new volume and that the previous volumes are available if requested.
- Test the human resources (HR) file system to ensure that access to the complete HR file is readily available (if the files are split and kept in two places or are located off-site). Review HR files and develop action plans for known deficient areas.
- Check stock supply of education materials and brochures on patient units, and ensure that they are available in English and other common languages for populations served by the organization.
- "Sweep" patient care units and departments for materials including outdated policies, procedures, guidelines, order sets, forms, and privilege binders.
- Check the environment to ensure that it is clean, including overlooked areas such as corners, ceiling tiles, and baseboards.
- Assign staff for command center duty and as escorts, scribes, and other roles. Determine both a primary and a back-up person for each role. The escort's primary function is to remain with the surveyor at all times so the surveyor is not unattended; escorts develop a relationship with an individual surveyor and should be consistent throughout the survey unless they are not a good match with the surveyor's personality. Escorts should be matched to surveyors with similar skill sets; for example, a physician with a physician or a nurse with a nurse. Scribes are responsible for documenting the activities of the surveyor and communicating directly with the command center as to those activities. Determine if confidentiality releases, security codes, access cards, or name badges will be needed and be sure escorts have access.
- If the organization is spread out over a geographic area, determine whether drivers are needed. Designate shuttle or transfer arrangements and drivers for surveyors to get to other locations. If employees are using their own vehicles, be sure vehicles are clean inside and out (consider arranging for a car detailing).
- Arrange for parking for surveyors. Designate spaces close to the main entrance; post "reserved for surveyors" signage during survey dates. If there is paid parking, be sure to provide surveyors with parking vouchers. Provide a facility map highlighting where the reserved parking is located. Consider also if there is a need to reserve parking spaces for employees driving surveyors.
- Distribute final survey schedules immediately prior to the survey and include surveyor names, if available. Consider enhancing schedules with room numbers/names, escort and scribe assignments, and names of participants assigned to each session.
- Ensure that the lead surveyor knows who the survey coordinator is, as this will be the person to contact for any information during the survey or in the evenings/weekends. Provide the survey coordinator's pager, cellular, and home phone numbers for after-hours or weekend issues.
- Prepare packets to be given to surveyors upon arrival. Include a map of the facility, facility contact list with phone numbers and pagers, organization chart, parking location map and parking voucher, guest ID badge, and survey agenda. Information or brochures on local area restaurants and attractions also may be appreciated.

3. Command Center

During a survey it is useful to have a central point of contact for surveyors and to manage and track all requests for information or interviews. The command center should have one person identified as being in charge; this often is the person identified as the organization's survey coordinator. The command center should be organized in advance with defined staff roles and should track key information including the surveyors and issues they identify, patients reviewed, charts requested, employees interviewed or files reviewed, physicians interviewed and involved in patient care, and surveyor requests.

- Determine how progress notes of requests will be kept and how information from escorts or scribes will be documented and shared with appropriate leaders and staff. The process should ensure closure of all issues during the survey. Tracking should include the responsible parties and status of the requests through closure.
- Discuss with surveyors in advance how they prefer to have information delivered to them. Consider a file or box for each individual surveyor's requests. Supplies such as chart pads, easels, grease boards, and clipboards may be used.
- Develop contact lists of key staff, managers, or departments. The command center will need phone numbers that are always answered for key departments, and the command center phone numbers will have to be published so that all staff involved in the survey know where to call.
- Consider distributing facsimile forms pre-addressed for the command center to all potential locations surveyors will visit to facilitate quick communication. These forms can also include the phone numbers, pager numbers, or cellular phone numbers for the command center.
- Specify the communication equipment that may have to be obtained specifically for this function. Many organizations have a room where this equipment is located permanently so that the room is ready for announced or unannounced survey operations, as well as for natural disasters. Determine the number of computers needed and ensure that active lines are available for mainframe computer access.
- Determine the amount of time needed to complete these requests far in advance and allow time to test equipment before the survey starts. Arrange for dedicated phone and facsimile lines. More than one phone line is required to allow open lines for return pages or call backs, and to allow more than one person to use the phone at a given time. One phone line should roll over to another line to eliminate busy signals.
- Make an administrative binder always available for any survey. This binder should include current organizational charts, program descriptions, plans for the provision of care, governing body structures, bylaws, current phone number lists, recent accreditation applications, and current copies of licenses. Consider also having a year of board of director minutes and key quality and administrative reports (such as scorecards and dashboards) readily available.

4. Survey Preparation Education

An education program for continuous readiness was discussed earlier. In addition to the topics described above, the following types of preparation should be considered for key staff involved in the planned survey:

- Review key standards as appropriate by department or functional area. Staff education booklets may be helpful for this process.
- Conduct orientation sessions for nursing unit charge nurses or departmental managers, physicians, and residents to help them understand their role and what to expect during the survey.
- Conduct orientation sessions for surveyor escorts and scribes: familiarize them with their role; provide tours of the facility to ensure that all escorts know the campus thoroughly and are aware of proper routes for guests; coach them to "tell the story" of things the organization is proud of (which might be triggered by things noted during the tour); and orient them to communication strategies with the command center.
- If orientation sessions will be held for the surveyors, conduct practice sessions with live audiences to enable the speakers to become familiar with the equipment, material, and questions that might come from the audience. Ensure that all managers and leaders attend the practice sessions so that they are aware of what will be highlighted.
- Practice known interviews with involved staff and include back-up personnel who may be called in at the last moment.
- Practice interviews with staff, focusing on questions such as "show me how…." or "show me where…"
- Review with senior leadership linkages with the governing body and how these are demonstrated through committee minutes.

5. Space Planning for Survey

Reserve all rooms required for survey activities as far in advance as possible to minimize the disruption caused when standing reservations need to be postponed, cancelled, or relocated during the survey. Prepare attendee lists for each activity to determine conference room sizes and set-up requirements. For any relocated or cancelled meetings, post the new room location on the door so survey meetings are not interrupted. Consider notifying enrolled participants when classes are moved or cancelled. All reserved survey rooms should be checked for set-up and working equipment daily during the survey.

Surveyors' workroom. Reserve a conference room for surveyors to work in privacy. This should be in a quiet location without other potentially noisy meetings in adjacent space. The room should be secure at night and when surveyors are out on clinical units. Set-up will require a workspace and chair for each surveyor, food service table, document table, telephone with speaker phone, and power source for all surveyor computers. It also may require one analog line or high-speed Internet line for surveyors to relay information to their organization's home office. This room will be used all day during every survey day and will not be available for other use in the evenings.

Survey command center room. Reserve a convenient location relative to the surveyor workroom. This room requires multiple tables or work spaces to accommodate chairs for staff use, food service, and documents. Arrange for the room to have at least two telephones and a facsimile machine, and at least two computers to allow rapid access to clinical systems and policies or procedures concurrently. This room will be used all day during every day of the survey and should not be available for use in the evenings by others, because this would require packing up confidential material daily. The room should be locked at night.

Other conference rooms to consider. If the survey schedule includes a daily briefing with surveyors or daily special issues resolution time, consider where to hold these sessions. Select a location that will comfortably hold anticipated participants away from surveyor workrooms or command center operations so that survey work is not interrupted. Consider also if the facility wishes to "huddle" with key staff, surveyor escorts or scribes, and leadership during lunch hours and at the beginning or end of the day. The facility may also wish to set a room aside for leadership strategy sessions during the survey process. At the end of the survey there is usually an exit conference, which will require chairs for staff and table and chairs for surveyors at the front of the room. Based on the number of anticipated participants, this could require a large conference room, in which case the need for microphones and audio recording equipment should be considered.

Additional hosting considerations relate to keeping staff and surveyors comfortable during the survey session. Order food daily for morning breakfast and lunch with delivery to the surveyors' workroom and the command center; in addition, the facility may wish to provide lunch for the management team involved in the survey. Make sure bottled water, coffee, tea, and snacks are available all day. It may be helpful to determine in advance if surveyors have special dietary needs or preferences. Remember to have rooms stocked daily with paper napkins, plates, utensils, and cups. Arrange with housekeeping for frequent trash removal after meals so that trash is not overflowing and food odor is not an issue. Identify key restrooms in advance that may have heavy use during the survey. Ensure that they are clean and in good repair and keep them stocked, which may require supplemental service schedules.

6. After the Survey

Even if the preliminary findings are favorable, there are still things the organization will need to do. It is very important to debrief as soon as possible after the survey. By the time of the closing conference, everyone is listening for those key final words, and critical information regarding potential recommendations in specific areas often is missed. This can be minimized, if following review of each aspect, the surveyors are asked to summarize findings. All notes taken during the survey should be reviewed and compared to comments made during the closing. The organization needs to be working on identified issues immediately. Responsibility for follow-up and completion of any written reports should be assigned to appropriate members of the team. Any areas not receiving substantial/significant compliance ratings should form the basis for future oversight agendas.

In addition, the team should evaluate the survey process, including the preparedness of management and staff in responding to questions; adequacy of documentation presentation; and flow of the survey process. Adjust the preparation process for future surveys accordingly. Should the team identify problems or issues with the survey team, responsibility for submission of a letter to the accrediting agency informing them of the specific complaint should be assigned. The CEO, chief of staff/medical director, and the chairman of the board should consider a special communication to all staff on the survey outcome and extend appreciation for their collaborative efforts.

The survey coordinator should make plans in advance for post-survey activities. Immediately after the survey, plan for a celebration to allow staff and managers to meet and celebrate completion of the survey (this will require a budget approved by leadership in advance). Plan for a leadership debriefing of survey findings immediately within days of the survey, while events are still fresh in participants' minds. Identify areas that will require action, and determine the process for corrective action plan development and oversight. Consider the need for committee approvals for work plan activities. Deadlines for responding to survey findings must be considered in the corrective action plan development.

I. Unannounced Visits or Survey Plans

Increasingly, accreditation and licensing agencies are conducting unannounced visits or surveys. Healthcare quality professionals should develop plans with leadership for how the organization will respond when an unannounced surveyor arrives. These plans facilitate a smooth survey regardless of who is present or available to assist the surveyor, as roles and expectations are understood in advance.

When surveyors arrive at a facility, they typically report to administrative offices and announce their visit. They may or may not present formal letters describing the reason for the visit. Administrative support staff should find a comfortable location for the surveyor to wait while the appropriate administrator is located. Support staff need to know whom to call when these situations arise (the designated administrator often is out of the office and their back-up needs to be identified quickly). After the administrator welcomes the surveyor, he or she must request to see a photo identification card from the represented agency or organization and obtain a business card from the surveyor (to ensure that contact information is available for any required follow-up). The survey should not proceed without proper surveyor identification.

The surveyor describes the purpose of the visit; this information should be used to assemble the appropriate team of individuals who have accountabilities related to the purpose of the visit. The surveyor may ask to visit departments or tour the facility, and they should be accompanied if at all possible. They may request to see copies of documents, review medical records, or review HR or credentialing files. Organizations should establish policies to guide staff as to what documents may be copied upon surveyor request and what documents need to be reviewed on-site.

During most surveys, the surveyor(s) conduct an exit conference prior to leaving the facility. This provides an opportunity for the organization to clarify findings or provide additional supporting information. Leadership should ask the surveyor to summarize the findings, including any violations or deficiencies that were noted; and to disclose anticipated next steps in the survey process, including any requirements for corrective action plans. If the surveyor does not leave a final report at the time of the survey, inquire as to the expected timeline for receipt of this important document. If deficiencies are suspected, the organization should develop and implement corrective actions immediately and not wait for a copy of the final report. If the final report is delayed, it may be difficult to remember details of the survey later when the report arrives, making corrective action planning more difficult. The organization also may be given a short deadline (10 days, for example) to submit corrective actions once the report is received.

V. Failure Mode and Effects Analysis (FMEA) for Readiness

Application of failure mode and effects analysis (FMEA) tools to proactively evaluate program plans for continuous readiness is a useful process to better understand where programs need to be strengthened, before they have an opportunity to fail and an organization experiences the consequences associated with noncompliance.

FMEA is a systematic method of identifying and preventing failures before they occur (McDermott, Mikulak, & Beauregard, 1996; Stamatis, 1995). Ideally, FMEAs are completed when a new system or redesign of a system is in the early stages of development, but also can be used on systems or processes that are already in place. For each *failure* identified (whether a known failure or a potential), an *analysis* is completed that determines the following: the way the process/subprocess step can fail to function or the manner in which the failure occurs (failure *mode*), the *effect* of the failure mode, and an estimate of the severity and probability for each mode-effect combination. An evaluation is completed as to what actions could be taken to reduce or eliminate the risk of the failure.

FMEA is one of many analytical tools that are part of the broad management practice of system readiness and safety. FMEA was used in the aerospace industry in the 1960s and has been a key safety tool in the chemical process industries (McDermott, et al., 1996). FMEA has received increased attention as healthcare begins to focus more on prevention of problems and attempts to proactively understand "what could go wrong" before it actually does. Historically, accident prevention has not been the primary focus of healthcare; instead, retrospective review has been used to examine data for events or outcomes that have already occurred. The Joint Commission added hospital leadership standards effective in July 2001 that required healthcare organizations to proactively address patient safety, using system safety tools like FMEA (Joint Commission, 2002; Joint Commission Resources, 2002). This standard was expanded to home healthcare programs in 2004.

Healthcare organizations have been working to create FMEA models that work in complex service environments (DeRosier, Stalhandske, Bagian, & Nudell, 2002). The Kaiser Permanente FMEA model was used to create a template for an FMEA to examine continuous readiness programs (Brown, Bonacum, & Vonderheide-Liem, 2005). This model was based on the work of McDermott et al. (1996), Stamatis (1995), and the Veterans Affairs National Center for Patient Safety (2001).

The following FMEA template can be used for proactive examination of "what could go wrong" with continuous readiness programs, before an organization experiences the associated consequences. A checklist to guide the process is provided in **Figure 3-4.**

Step 1. Define the FMEA boundaries.

Most teams will want to use the FMEA Team Start-up Worksheet (**Figure 3-5**) to organize and document the FMEA process in addition to using tools from existing performance improvement models to document the improvement actions taken. The FMEA leadership sponsors and the FMEA team leader must work together to plan the FMEA project. The team conducting the analysis will need an overview of the existing or proposed continuous readiness program. Useful documents to assemble would be charters for oversight committees, work plans, and any readiness project management documents that exist.

Step 2. Assemble the FMEA team.

FMEA is a team function. The purpose of the FMEA team is to bring a variety of perspectives and experiences to the project. FMEA teams are specifically defined for an individual project, are cross-functional and multidisciplinary, and may disband after the FMEA project is completed. The continuous readiness program leader and key stakeholders should be identified as key team members for this analysis. An impartial facilitator should be identified rather than assigning facilitation to key stakeholders or process owners who have designed the existing program.

Figure 3-4. Kaiser Permanente Model: Failure Mode and Effects Analysis (FMEA) Checklist Applied to Continuous Readiness Programs

Date Started ________	**Team Leader** ________
Step 1: Define the FMEA Boundaries	• Describe the continuous readiness program and the FMEA boundaries. • Define individual and team responsibilities.
Step 2: Assemble the FMEA Team	• Assign team leader and ensure adequate team composition. • Complete the "FMEA Team Start-up Worksheet."
Step 3: Review the Process	• Flowchart the continuous readiness program. • Number process and subprocess steps.
Step 4: Brainstorm Potential Failure Modes	• Determine all the ways each process/subprocess step could fail.
Step 5: Identify the Potential Cause(s) of Each Failure Mode	• Identifying potential cause(s) at this point provides some insight into probability.
Step 6: List Potential Effects on the Patient	• For each failure mode, identify potential effects.
Step 7: Assign Risk Codes	• Assign a risk code (from the risk matrix) to each potential failure-mode effect combination. • As likelihood or probability requires an "exposure interval" to be decided, it may be easiest to think of a survey cycle when thinking about the likelihood of harm.
Step 8: Develop Actions or Countermeasures to Reduce Risk	• Identify countermeasures (e.g., feasible actions, controls) to reduce or eliminate the risk associated with the failure mode.
Step 9: Re-assign Risk Codes (Residual Risk)	• With each recommended action, determine what the risk code would become after implementation (this is called the "residual risk"). • This code will assist in prioritizing actions and monitoring to determine if the actions were effective in reducing risk.
Step 10: Assign Responsibility for Actions	• Assign responsibility for implementing corrective actions and determine project completion date.
Step 11: Monitor the Actions and Risk Reduction	• Monitor to evaluate if the risk reduction strategies have reduced risk. • Take additional action, if necessary, to further reduce risk.

Source: Brown, Bonacum, & Vonderheide-Leim, 2005.

Step 3. Review the process.

To ensure that everyone on the FMEA team has the same understanding of the process under investigation, review the process by creating a detailed flowchart of the existing or planned continuous readiness program. It may be useful to flowchart key survey cycles (e.g., a 2- or 3-year accreditation program process, perhaps selecting the most critical program) with process steps for continuous readiness linked to milestones in the survey cycle. Develop the flowchart as a

Figure 3-5. FMEA Team Start-up Worksheet (FMEA Steps 1 and 2)

Kaiser Facility:		Date FMEA Started:	
FMEA Project Name:			
Team Leader:		Team Sponsors:	
Team Members: (Step 2)	♦ ♦ ♦		♦ ♦ ♦

Team Leader Questions:

1. Are all affected areas represented?	Yes No If No, Actions:
2. Are different levels and types of knowledge represented on the team?	Yes No If No, Actions:
3. Who will maintain the records?	

FMEA Team Project Boundaries (Step 1):

1. Project Purpose (including a brief description of the process under review):	
2. What aspects of the FMEA is the team responsible for?	❑ FMEA Analysis ❑ Recommendations for Improvement ❑ Implementation of Improvements
3. Reporting Body(s): Who will receive progress reports?	
4. Project Deadlines:	
5. What is the process if the team needs to expand beyond these boundaries?	

Source: Brown, Bonacum, & Vonderheide-Liem, 2005.

team—for example, using self-sticking notes on a wall or board, until the process is agreed upon—then transfer the diagram into a permanent document for future reference. Transcribe process steps onto the FMEA Team Worksheet (**Figure 3-6**) and use this worksheet for Steps 4 through 9 (FMEA Step 3 is carried over on the worksheet to help keep the team organized).

Step 4. Brainstorm potential failure modes.

Once the team has an understanding of the process, the next step is to determine all the ways each readiness process step could fail (failure modes). Brainstorming should include a review related to categories such as people, methods, equipment, materials, and the environment of the process; also consider policies (high-level decision rules) and procedures (steps in a task). Focusing on each of the categories will result in a more thorough list of potential failure modes.

Step 5. Identify the potential cause(s) of each failure mode.

Potential causes of the failure mode can provide insight into the probability of failure and direct the team toward prevention and/or corrective actions. The more focused the FMEA is on the causes, the more successful the team will be in eliminating potential failures. Try to answer the question, "What most likely could cause the failure?"

Step 6. List the potential effects.

For each failure mode listed on the FMEA team worksheet, identify the potential effects of the failure should it occur. The effect is the outcome—try to answer the questions, "What happens when a failure occurs?" or "What is(are) the consequence(s)?" or "If this happens, then what happens to the patient?"

Step 7. Assign risk codes.

Next, the team evaluates the severity and likelihood of each failure mode-effect combination on the organization. This step of the FMEA attempts to assign risk codes to all potential failure mode-effect combinations so that they can be prioritized for actions to reduce or eliminate them.

Figure 3-6. Failure Mode and Effects Analysis Worksheet

FMEA Project Title : Medical Center: Date:								
FMEA Step 3	*FMEA Step 4*	*FMEA Step 5*	*FMEA Step 6*	*FMEA Step 7*			*FMEA Step 8*	*FMEA Step 9*
Process Step	Failure Modes	Potential Causes	Potential Effects	Likelihood or Probability of Harm	Severity of Harm Level	Risk Code or Number	Recommended Actions and Countermeasures	Residual Risk Code After Action

Source: Brown, Bonacum, & Vonderheide-Liem, 2005.

Likelihood of harm is the probability of this failure occurring during an exposure interval. Defining an exposure interval can be done in many ways, but thinking of a period of one survey cycle may be most beneficial (e.g., a 2- or 3-year accreditation program process, perhaps selecting the most critical program). *Severity of harm* is an estimation of how serious the effects or harm would be if a given failure did occur. In some cases, it is clearly based on past experience. In other cases, it is necessary to estimate the severity of a failure mode based on the knowledge and expertise of the team members. Because each failure may have several different effects and each effect can have a different level of severity, it is the effect, not the failure, that is rated. The team should determine the likelihood of the worst credible outcome and the worst credible severity of harm by using the FMEA team risk-assessment matrix (**Figure 3-7**). *Worst credible* is a reasonable worst case, not the worst conceivable case.

Step 8. Develop actions or countermeasures to reduce risks.

Next, the team identifies feasible actions (controls or countermeasures) to eliminate or reduce the high-risk failure modes. The team will want to prioritize for action plan development those effects that create the highest risk for the organization related to survey readiness.

Step 9. Reassign risk codes (residual risk).

With each recommended action, determine what the risk code would become after implementation of the planned actions. This is a theoretical exercise that involves the team's best judgments. The theoretical risk remaining if the planned actions were completed is the *residual risk*. Residual risk scores help the team carefully examine the planned actions to determine if additional actions should be developed.

Step 10. Assign responsibility for actions.

It is important to assign responsibility and target the completion date. The continuous readiness leadership or oversight group should provide ongoing oversight to ensure the follow-up needed for a successful readiness program.

Step 11. Monitor the action results and risk reduction.

Once the actions have been implemented, the team or group assigned accountability for the actions should continue to document the FMEA actions as part of the FMEA documentation. The monitoring plan should include data to evaluate the result of actions when possible, or data to determine if new risks have been introduced with process changes. The FMEA team action/countermeasure worksheet (**Figure 3-8**) will facilitate this documentation.

Figure 3-7. FMEA Team Risk-Assessment Matrix

			Likelihood of Harm (Probability) (During one survey cycle)					
		Level	F	E	D	C	B	A
		Description	Impossible	Improbable	Remote	Occasional	Probable	Frequent
		Definition	Physically impossible to occur	So unlikely it can be assumed occurrence may not be experienced	Not likely to occur but possible during survey cycle	May occur in/during survey cycle	Quite likely to occur in/ during survey cycle	Occurrence almost certain in/during survey cycle
Likelihood of Harm (Probability)	I. Catastrophic	Loss of license or accreditation	3	3	2	1	1	1
	II. Critical	Notice of termination; extensive adverse media; extensive corrective actions required	3	3	3	2	1	1
	III. Marginal	Corrective actions required	3	3	3	3	2	2
	IV. Negligible	Identification of improvement opportunities	3	3	3	3	3	3

Risk Codes

High-Risk	1	Medium-Risk	2	Low-Risk	3

Source: Brown, Bonacum, & Vonderheide-Liem, 2005.

Figure 3-8. Failure Mode and Effects Analysis Action/Countermeasure Worksheet

FMEA Project Title :
Medical Center:
Date:

FMEA Step 3	*FMEA Step 4*	*FMEA Step 8*	*FMEA Step 9*	*FMEA Step 10*		*FMEA Step 11*	*FMEA Step 11*	
Process Step	Failure modes	Recommended Actions and Countermeasures	Residual Risk Code or number After Action	Responsible Person	Target Completion Date	Monitoring of Action Results	Action Completion Date	Recalculated Residual Risk Code

Source: Brown, Bonacum, & Vonderheide-Liem, 2005.

VI. Summary

This module began with reflection of recent survey experiences that may have been representative of cultures of cyclic survey preparation, just-in-time training, and crisis management. Throughout the module, tools have been provided to help healthcare quality professionals begin the journey to create a culture of continuous readiness to meet public expectations for safe patient care at all times, that is, not cyclic and minimizing crisis management. Healthcare quality professionals can begin to think of their organizations using the framework of complex adaptive systems and to apply management principles that may be very different than previous ones. The Eight-Stage Process of Creating Continuous Readiness in Complex Organizations can guide those leading this cultural change. The key components of successful readiness programs can be evaluated to prioritize infrastructure improvements as well as organizational culture. Survey preparation processes can guide leadership through planning for a successful survey process. And the FMEA tools can be used to proactively evaluate readiness programs before they have the opportunity to fail and organizations experience noncompliance consequences.

References

Brown, D.S., Bonacum, D., & Vonderheide-Liem, D. (2005). The Kaiser Permanente FMEA Model: Simplified for healthcare personnel. *Journal for Healthcare Quality, 27*(1), 48–55.

Cameron, K. (1995). Downsizing, quality, and performance. In R.E. Cole (Ed.), *The fall and rise of the American quality movement*. New York: Oxford University Press.

Cameron, K.S., & Ettington, D.R. (1988). The conceptual foundations of organizational culture. In *Higher education: Handbook of theory and research*, pp. 356–396. New York: Agathon.

Cameron, K.S., Freeman, S.J., & Mishra, A.K. (1991). Best practices in white-collar downsizing: Managing contradictions. *Academy of Management Executive, 5*, 57–73.

Cameron, K.S., & Quinn, R.E. (1999). *Diagnosing and changing organizational culture: Based on the competing values framework.* New York: Addison Wesley.

Daniels, W.R., & Mathers, J.G. (1997). *Change-ABLE organization: Key management practices for speed and flexibility*. Mill Valley, CA: ACT Publishing.

DeRosier, J., Stalhandske, E., Bagian, J.P., & Nudell, T. (2002). Using healthcare failure mode and effects analysis: The VA National Center for Patient Safety's Prospective Risk Analysis System. *The Joint Commission Journal on Quality Improvement, 28*(5), 248–267.

Joint Commission on Accreditation of Healthcare Organizations. (2002). *2002 hospital accreditation standards.* Oakbrook Terrace, IL: Joint Commission Resources.

Joint Commission Resources. (2002). *Failure mode and effects analysis in healthcare: Proactive risk reduction.* Oakbrook Terrace, IL: Author.

Kotter, J.P. (1996). *Leading change.* Boston: Harvard Business School Press.

Kozlowski, S., Chao, G.T., Smith, E.M., & Hedlund, J. (1993). Organizational downsizing: Strategies, interventions, and research implications. *International Review of Industrial and Organizational Psychology, 8*, 263–332.

McDermott, R.E., Mikulak, R.J., & Beauregard, M. (1996). *The basics of FMEA*. Portland, OR: Productivity, Inc.

Merriam-Webster Online Dictionary. [Online.] Retrieved May 23, 2005, from http://www.m-w.com/

O'Toole, J.O. (1996). *Leading change: The argument for values-based leadership*. New York: Ballantine Books.

Plsek, P.E. (2001). Redesigning healthcare with insights from the science of complex adaptive systems. In Committee on Quality of Healthcare in America, Institute of Medicine. Appendex B in *Crossing the quality chasm: A new health system for the 21st century.* Washington: National Academies Press.

Plsek, P.E. (2004, June). *The door into summer: Transformational change in complex systems.* Keynote address at 2004 Kaiser Permanente National Quality Conference, "Riding the Wave: Creativity, Innovation, Courage," San Diego, CA.

Plsek, P.E., & Kilo, C.M. (1999). From resistance to attraction: A different approach to change. *Physician Executive, 25*(6), 40–46.

Stamatis, D.H. (1995). *Failure mode and effects analysis: FMEA from theory to execution.* Milwaukee, WI: American Society for Quality.

Veterans Affairs National Center for Patient Safety. (2001). *The basics of healthcare failure mode and effects analysis.* Retrieved May 25, 2005, from http://www.va.gov/ncps

Zimmerman, B., Lindberg, C., & Plsek, P. (2001). *Edgeware: Insights from complexity science for healthcare leaders.* Irving, TX: VHA, Inc.

Suggested Reading

Brown, S.L., & Eisenhardt, K.M. (1998). *Competing on the edge: Strategy as structured chaos.* Boston: Harvard Business School Press.

Fraser, S.W., & Greenhalgh, T. (2001). Complexity science: Coping with complexity, educating for capability. *British Medical Journal, 323*, 799–803.

Greenhalgh, T., & Plsek, P.E. (2001). Four-part special series on complex science. *British Medical Journal, 323*, 625–628.

Holland, J.H. (1998). *Emergence: From chaos to order*. Reading, MA: Helix Books.

Johnson, B. (1996). *Polarity management: Identifying and managing unsolvable problems.* Amherst, MA: HRD Press.

Peters, T. (1987). *Thriving on chaos*. New York: Knopf.

Plsek, P.E., & Greenhalgh, T. (2001). The challenge of complexity in healthcare. *British Medical Journal, 323*, 625–628.

Schein, E. H. (2004). *Organization culture and leadership*. San Francisco: Jossey Bass.

Simmons, A. (2002). *The story factor: Inspiration, influence, and persuasion through the art of storytelling*. New York: Basic Books.

Stacey, R.D. (1996). *Complexity and creativity in organizations*. San Francisco: Berrett-Koehler Publishers.

Waldrop, M.M. (1992). *Complexity: The emerging science at the edge of order and chaos*. New York: Simon & Schuster.

Wilson, T., & Holt, T. (2001). Complexity science: Complexity and clinical care. *British Medical Journal, 323*, 685–688.

MODULE FOUR

Change Management and Innovation

Susan V. White, PhD RN CPHQ FNAHQ

"It is not the strongest of the species that survive, nor the most intelligent, but the ones most responsive to change." Charles Darwin

I. Introduction

Within the healthcare environment, change is not only inevitable but also an ingredient essential for growth. Without change, there would be stagnation within systems and new knowledge and technology would not be adopted. Change is constant and occurs at all levels of healthcare organizations. Each level of change requires different strategies, depending on

- the type of change
- the people involved
- the magnitude of the behavior that must be modified to make the required change.

The ability to manage change in a planned, productive manner is a key skill often needed by healthcare quality professionals. Therefore, it is necessary to understand various aspects of change, change models, and how to use tools to successfully manage change for improvement. This section provides an overview of the key concepts associated with change, models that describe how change occurs, strategies to manage change, and tools to help accelerate successful change.

Healthcare is a complex system in which demands change quickly. There is intense competition among various healthcare organizations, and this competition is intensified due to limited resources. The question facing most organizations is not whether they should make changes, but rather how much and how often. Two factors are critical to assessing change in organizations: the first factor to assess is the limits of human performance in being able to respond to change; the second factor is the actual capacity of the systems to handle change. An organization's ability to handle frequent change is largely dependent upon the individuals within the organization, including its leaders. The resiliency of individuals is a critical element in an organization's ability to make changes quickly and to rebound from one change to the next. While individual resiliency will have an effect on an organization's response to change, the leaders establish the culture of change, role model flexibility, and the behaviors needed to adapt to change.

"Resilience is the process of adapting well in the face of adversity, trauma, tragedy, threats, or even significant sources of stress—such as family and relationship problems, serious health problems, or workplace and financial stressors" (American Psychological Association [APA], 2003, paragraph 1). The APA recommends that individuals follow these guidelines to build and sustain resilience:

- make connections (good relationships)
- avoid seeing crises as insurmountable problems
- accept that change is a part of living
- move toward goals
- take decisive actions
- look for opportunities for self-discovery
- nurture a positive self-view
- keep things in perspective
- maintain a hopeful outlook
- take care of self.

Often, change is distinguished either as "first-order change" or "second-order change." First-order change involves small, relatively easy steps and requires minimal effort to achieve. It rarely has a significant effect on systems or organizations. For example, a first-order change might be a new form or pickup time or the same product with a new vendor. Second-order change, however, is complex and requires a significant change in behavior to achieve desired new ways of performing new processes. For example, a second-order change might be implementing a new computer or new clinical guidelines or restricting a formulary. This is important to understand at the outset, as change requires energy, effort, and work. Because people often underestimate both the amount of work and the time required to implement change, a well-designed plan should include sufficient resources and time frames to complete each step in a plan.

Change is intrinsically linked with how people view their work processes and how much commitment they have invested in the current method of work or status quo. Change of a significant magnitude often entails loss of emotional comfort and may cause distress. While learning a new routine often is not hard, it is very difficult to "unlearn" or forget old habits. It can be easy to revert to the status quo or original ways of behaving, if methods are not implemented to sustain the change.

Although change generally is focused on moving people from an existing state through a transition state to a future state, no single conceptual model is useful in all change situations. People will be influenced by others and by interpersonal interactions as they move through the change process. This type of change is best managed by focusing on each person involved in the change process at the same time that the overall change is occurring within the organization. This is important because the final success of any change will be based on the perceptions of and acceptance by the people involved in the change.

If participants view the change as positive, they are more likely to value the results. On the other hand, if they are not part of the change process, they probably will not accept the changes that result; this will be evident in several ways. Commonly, disgruntled staff will return to the old way of practice. They may devise work-around solutions or outright sabotage in order to avoid the change. Healthcare quality professionals play vital roles as change agents, improvement advisors, and facilitators and must be attuned to the personal side of change in order to manage the change process successfully. Healthcare is in constant flux, and the success of healthcare organizations in the future will depend on their flexibility and implementation of change in a routine manner.

One of the most important change concepts to understand is that "All changes do not necessarily lead to improvement, but all improvement requires change" (Institute for Healthcare Improvement [IHI], "How to Improve" [n.d., paragraph 6]). People may make changes that have no impact on improving services or products, but that will certainly disrupt routines. This must be clearly understood by healthcare quality professionals because of the turmoil and upheaval that constant change creates for day-to-day workflow. When change improves services and products, it is easier for healthcare quality professionals and other members of the change team to positively influence those who must make the change. Change merely for the sake of change usually causes frustration and dissatisfaction, not to mention additional work.

No single model or tool will fit every situation in which change is desired. A repertoire of skills and knowledge will help healthcare quality professionals to understand different views of how change occurs and to use a variety of tools and techniques to effectively manage change. A number of change models that describe how change occurs, as well as some change management strategies based on their theoretical frameworks, are presented.

II. Change Models

A. Lewin's Change Model

Kurt Lewin had a strong impact on the theory and practice of social and organizational psychology. Of particular interest is his change model, the first premise of which is that motivation and readiness for change must occur before the change can actually take place. The impetus to change is based on a "force field" of driving and restraining forces. For change to occur, the force field must be altered so that driving forces are stronger than restraining forces. A key concept of Lewin's model is that the force field—and therefore the impetus to change—could be affected more by removing restraining forces than by adding more driving force. To create the motivation to change, there has to be some level of frustration or dissatisfaction with the current situation. This dissatisfaction creates a level of anxiety or creative tension that will spur the desire to change. Effective change managers will use the dissatisfaction with the status quo to begin the movement to change.

This first step in Lewin's change process, known as "unfreezing," means that beliefs, expectations, and norms can be remolded into new beliefs and behaviors. Through a process of learning new information, attitudes, and processes, people are able to redefine their current beliefs and "refreeze" these new concepts into their behaviors. This model is useful in approaching change in behaviors and identifying strategies to accelerate change and sustain new desired behaviors.

Models of change typically show movement from a current state or old system to a new or future state. This involves first unfreezing or changing the old system and moving it out of a "comfort zone" so that change can occur. This progresses to a transition state or middle ground, through which the now unfrozen process is altered. Finally, a new system or future state of equilibrium emerges. This new state must be refrozen so the new change "sticks." This model has been used to integrate human system change with technology and work systems changes. It also can be used to create new systems to foster new activities needed by redesigned or reengineered work processes. The focus of the change effort is to invent a new status quo by directing all the activities and people involved in the change process (Accel-team, 2004; Schein, n.d; Smith, 2004).

Figure 4-1 depicts the change model of moving from a current state by unfreezing behavior, through the transition state, and, finally, to a future state by refreezing a new behavior.

Figure 4-1. Unfreezing/Refreezing Model

Current State	Transition State	Future State
Unfreeze old behavior	Intervening change	Refreeze new behavior

The tool that can be used to analyze a situation or process to be changed, based on Lewin, is force field analysis (see **Figure 4-2**). A diagram of two columns—"driving" and "restraining" forces—is developed to analyze opposing forces related to a specific change. Brainstorming, in a verbal format, and brainwriting, in a written format, are tools that can be used to identify the driving and restraining forces if they are not readily apparent. Driving forces, such as incentives and competition, tend to push change in a particular direction and keep it going.

Figure 4-2. Force Field Analysis Tool

Driving Forces	Restraining Forces
→	←
→	←
Example: Proposed change is to add music therapy as an adjunct therapy for pain management in oncology patients on the oncology unit.	
Recommendation by the National Comprehensive Cancer Network Guidelines to add music therapy and/or diversion therapy as an adjunct to pain management therapies. →	Music therapy requires additional documentation by the nursing staff and there is no place to document this intervention in the current computer record. ←
Support by the clinical nurse specialist on the oncology unit. →	There is a cost for CD equipment and CDs, which is not covered in the current budget. ←
Research on music therapy in oncology patients provides support that it increases relaxation and perception of pain relief by patients. →	There is an increase in job responsibilities for the person who must manage the CDs, equipment, and library of music. ←
Alternative therapies are commonly used by patients at home. →	Equipment must be tracked because it can be easily removed from the unit, increasing losses and therefore costs. ←
	Staff knowledge and philosophy of pain management are based on a traditional model with little knowledge about alternative forms of pain management. ←
Example: Proposed change is to allow families 24-hour visiting hours for patients in the intensive care unit.	
Families provide comfort and reassurance to patients during ICU stays. Long periods without family support may increase stress. →	Medical director finds the open visiting policy disruptive to patient care. ←
Patients have a right to have family present during illness. →	Nursing staff finds the open visiting policy disruptive to nursing routines and getting their work done. ←
Families have variable work schedules and cannot always meet the hospital's schedule. →	The open visiting hours will tire patients and not allow sufficient rest. ←
	More families will stay overnight and crowd waiting rooms, sleeping on chairs and couches. ←
	More families in the hospital throughout the night increase security risks for the hospital. ←

Restraining forces, which might include apathy or hostility, tend to restrain or decrease the driving forces. For change to be possible, the driving forces must be greater than the restraining forces. However, the force field analysis shows not only the number of opposing forces, but also the significance of each force. It is useful, for clarity, to indicate the relative "weights" of the opposing forces with the size of arrows (Figure 4-2). For example, if a new law requires that a particular change be made, this mandate, together with the threat of a large fine for noncompliance, would be a more powerful driving force than would a manager's lack of interest in the particular change (the lack of money could also be a strongly weighted restraining force).

A key change management strategy using the force field analysis is to reduce the number of restraining forces; this approach increases the chances of success. Note, however, that adding powerful drivers does not necessarily make change happen faster.

B. Palmer's Change Model

Another change model, by Palmer, uses seven key elements describing change from a current state, through a transition state, to an improved future state similar to Lewin's model. The change model elements described by Palmer are listed and then illustrated in **Figure 4-3**.

1. Leading change
2. Creating a shared need
3. Shaping a vision
4. Mobilizing commitment
5. Monitoring progress
6. Finishing the job
7. Anchoring the change in systems and structure (Palmer, 2004)

Figure 4-3. Change Model

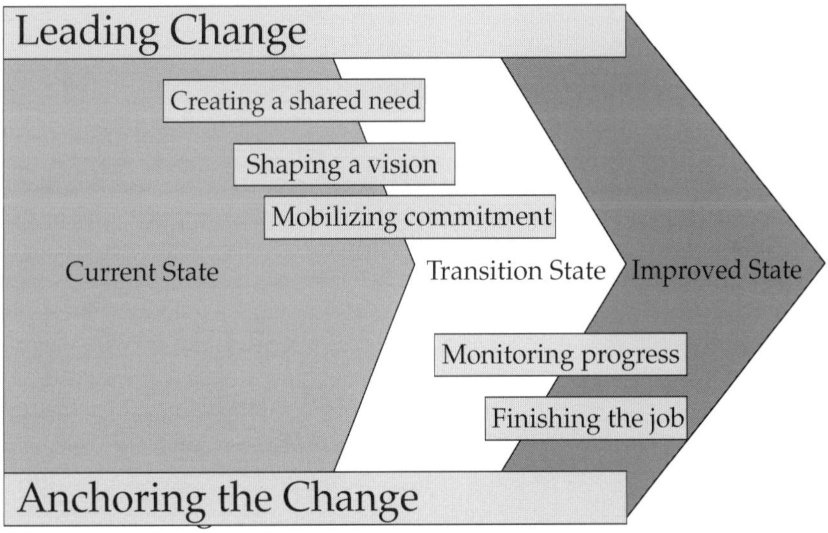

Reprinted with permission from Making change work: Practical tools for overcoming human resistance to change *by Brien Palmer. © 2004, ASQ Quality Press, Milwaukee, WI.*

The elements in **Table 4-1** will assist in assessing failure points and the needed change element for success using Palmer's model.

A key strategy to manage change using Palmer's model is to first assess "readiness." By using the change readiness guidelines listed in **Table 4-2**, an organization's readiness for change can be assessed. If the elements accompanying the change readiness guidelines do not indicate organizational readiness, then strategies should be developed to create readiness.

Palmer (2004a; 2004b) further describes how to assess readiness using the guidelines (Table 4-2). To use the tool, follow these instructions:

Table 4-1. Change Elements Necessary for Success

Change Model Element	Consequence of Missing a Model Element
Leading change	Change is slow, lacks attention and resources.
Creating a shared need	Change has a low priority; receives no attention; and starts, then stops.
Shaping a vision	Change gets off to a fast start that fizzles; there is no clear direction.
Mobilizing commitment	Nobody "owns" the change; the project is not sustainable.
Monitoring progress	There is no chance for feedback and improvement.
Finishing the job	Cynicism, naysaying, and a "fad-of-the-month" attitude abound.
Anchoring the change	Mixed signals, anxiety, and frustration increase.

Reprinted with permission from Making change work: Practical tools for overcoming human resistance to change *by Brien Palmer. © 2004, ASQ Quality Press, Milwaukee, WI.*

1. Use Table 4-2 to assess readiness in each of the categories listed and identify the corresponding percentage (e.g., if no one is in charge, then this would rate as 10%).
2. After each category has been assessed, add the first three categories. If the sum of categories 1 + 2 + 3 < 50%, then the likelihood of success for the change is low and even starting a project is risky. Consider delaying the change project until support is garnered.
3. If any single category is rated <50%, then the likelihood of success is also low (e.g., if no one is in charge, then chances of success are slim).
4. If the sum of categories 6 + 7 < 50%, then proceeding with a change to a successful change is unlikely.
5. The greater the percentage of readiness for change, the greater the likelihood of success. This approach also demonstrates the interrelatedness of each factor for change; all elements are important.
6. Plotting the percentage of readiness by each category helps visualize the state of readiness and consider strategies for various stages of the change project and the critical elements at different points.

C. DeWeaver and Gillespie's Change Model

Most change models used in healthcare are based on a perception that assumes the change process can be broken into component parts (a reductionist approach), and then healthcare quality professionals objectively measure the system inputs and outputs for each part. This model is most useful when there are objective measures, to predict accurate results. It depends on an orderly system, in which objects behave in predictable ways and new information can fit into existing structures (DeWeaver & Gillespie, 1997).

The following is a breakdown of the stages within this change model described by DeWeaver and Gillespie (1997):

- *Awareness stage*—The person knows something or is aware of the change and may have heard it mentioned before and explained. However, the individual generally does not have a strong opinion about it, or even denies that the change will affect him or her.
- *Curiosity stage*—The person expresses concern or curiosity, or asks questions about the effect of the change on him or her, and may be defensive, resistant, or in denial about the change.

Table 4-2. Change Readiness Guidelines

Category	10% Readiness	50% Readiness	90% Readiness
1. Leading change	No one is in charge.	Leader is pretty clear; management commitment is clear in some areas.	There is a clear sponsor, clear management commitment, no doubt.
2. Creating shared need	Most people are happy with the status quo.	Many people think a change is needed.	Everybody knows a change is needed.
3. Shaping a vision	What vision?	There is some consensus on what is needed, but also some apathy.	Everyone knows the needed outcome.
4. Mobilizing commitment	A staffer might help someone.	There are some resources dedicated, but more are needed to finish the job.	All the needed dedicated resources are available.
5. Monitoring progress	Everyone has their own opinion.	Some things are measured, but staff also go by gut feeling sometimes.	There are clear metrics for every activity being performed.
6. Finishing the job	Looks like a "dump and run."	Some plans have been made, but there is more to do.	There has been a pilot run, training, and recognition; everyone is ready.
7. Anchoring the change	Why does anything have to be done?	Discussion about this has begun, but hasn't really finished.	Everyone knows exactly what to adjust to embed this change.

- *Visualization stage*—The person now seeks to understand the relationship and the effect of the change on him or her, or on the organization as a whole, by asking questions and seeking information.
- *Learning stage*—The person takes part in learning how to implement or use the change and may offer opinions and concerns about specifics of the change.
- *Use stage*—The person actively uses the change and integrates the change into his or her daily work habits and can describe or explain the change to others (DeWeaver & Gillespie, 1997).

Individuals progress through these stages at different rates and can revert to previous stages at any time. Because the model is not linear, some people never make it through all of the stages. The change agent can't force people into later stages if they have not dealt with earlier stages. Whatever actions the facilitator does to assist people through the change process will need to be repeated many times for various groups of people. Some individuals may need the same process repeated several times. Others will need more time and more examples of benefits before they commit to a change (DeWeaver & Gillespie, 1997). This is commonly known as "What's in it for me?"

There are specific strategies for each stage of the change model, to increase the speed of the change process: awareness, curiosity, visualization, learning, and use.

- *Awareness stage*—Advertising in various media is used to inform people that the change is coming. Take the opportunity to highlight the positive effects of the change, and link the change to meeting staff needs and eliminating problems. Increasing awareness about the change early on provides an opportunity to shape perceptions positively.
- *Curiosity stage*— Strategies for the curiosity stage include providing frequent, clear, concise explanations and answering all questions. Taking time to elicit staff concerns and acknowledge the difficulties that the change may or will cause engenders support later in the change process. At the same time, it is important to present a viable approach to the change that acknowledges staff concerns. The curiosity stage is the time to create a level of dissatisfaction with the status quo and to generate interest in a new approach.
- *Visualization stage*—The strategy is to demonstrate the change for people and conduct user testing and reviews of the proposed changes. This strategy is further explained in Section VI Spread of Change and Innovation: Rogers' Diffusion Model; this is when the people implementing the change have an opportunity to try the change before it is put into place.
- *Learning stage*—This should focus on educating staff regarding the change. This stage includes conducting workshops or training sessions for as many staff members as possible, and giving them the opportunity for hands-on involvement when appropriate. Additional strategies include providing materials that will make the change easier to use, such as quick reference guides, troubleshooting tips, or "help" desks.
- *Use stage*—Technical assistance may be needed to make the change happen efficiently and effectively, with enough resources to enable people to become experts at the change.

All the users will be at different stages of accepting and implementing the change. Early in the change process, facilitators should meet with all stakeholder groups to communicate the change, especially discussing the rationale as to why it is needed at that particular time. They should take time to elicit reactions to the change, and be sure to correct any misunderstandings. Also, it is important to acknowledge people's reactions to the changes and ask for suggestions that will help overcome any obstacles. In summary, key strategies include multiple approaches to garner support for the change and keep people informed of the change process.

As the change is being implemented, it is important to continually assess the degree of its acceptance by the staff. This requires observing people's behavior and noting responses. Then, it is necessary to determine the stage of the change process in which people are operating. People will use many different methods to demonstrate resistance to change, and some may try to actually sabotage the change. Reengineering change projects frequently do not have a good success rate (DeWeaver & Gillespie, 1997). It will be necessary to find ways to help people identify with the change and understand it, and also to deal with their concerns. For change to succeed in an organization, a critical mass must support the new change.

People tend to fall into three groups related to change: those who are for change, those against the change, and those who are undecided. If efforts are focused on individuals who are already positively disposed to the change, they can in turn encourage those who are undecided, thereby allowing the facilitator to amass critical support. At this point, the focus should turn to individuals who are not supportive, so that they can be influenced to accept the change.

Early in the change process, a communication plan must be developed to ensure that everyone becomes aware of the changes that will occur. This may be easier to accomplish by envisioning concerns that people may have and proactively addressing them. This can be achieved by providing a forum in which individuals can express their concerns honestly. Any forums should involve supportive stakeholders early in a demonstration of the change, and should include enough time for people to deal with their emotions regarding the change and to help them let go of the past and embrace the future (DeWeaver & Gillespie, 1997).

To summarize, key strategies that a change agent can use to accelerate change using this model include

- assessing change readiness
- leading the change process proactively
- creating a shared need with stakeholders
- shaping a vision with clear goals
- mobilizing commitment with those who support the change
- monitoring progress toward completion
- completing the job
- anchoring the change in systems and structures.

D. Galpin's Human Side of Change Model

Traditional views of change claim that most organizations have focused on the technical, financial, and operational aspects, with little regard for the human aspect (Galpin, 1996b). This mindset has now shifted to a strong appreciation of the human side of change. After all, people do the work, people must make the changes, and people will support or resist the changes. Galpin's approach is based on a nine-step process in which change is a deliberate planned process. Having a well-planned, well thought-out process is the best approach to change management. Except in unusual circumstances, planning for change, rather than allowing it to occur haphazardly, will ensure the greatest degree of success.

Galpin's change management model involves the following steps:

- establish the need to change
- develop and disseminate a vision of the change
- diagnose/analyze the current situation
- generate goals and recommendations
- detail recommendations
- pilot-test recommendations
- prepare recommendations for rollout/spread
- understand and communicate the changes
- roll out/spread the changes throughout the desired units/organization
- measure, reinforce, and refine changes
- provide feedback
- offer rewards and recognition.

These steps are incorporated in **Figure 4-4**. Galpin correlates these stages with suggested time frames to guide the facilitator in planning, and also correlates the stages with either strategic change or grassroots change. Strategic change involves stages 1, 2, 3, 4, and 5 and grassroots change involves stages 6, 7, 8, and 9. Teams are basic infrastructure for the use of this model (Galpin, 1996b).

Figure 4-4. Change Management Process Model

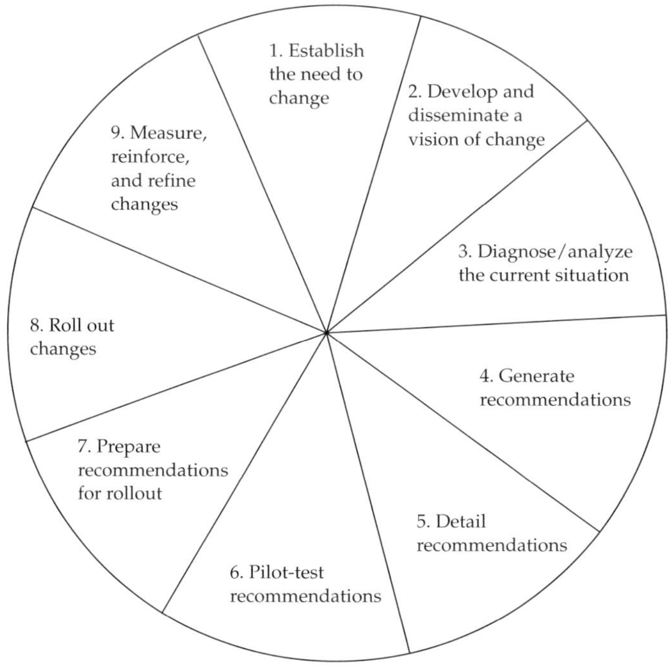

Source: The Human Side of Change *by Timothy J. Galpin, © 1996, Jossey-Bass Publishers, San Francisco. Reprinted with permission of John Wiley & Sons, Inc.*

Using his nine-step model, Galpin identifies four communication phases of a change effort. First is the "build awareness" phase (corresponds to stages 1 and 2). Next is the "project status" phase (corresponds to stages 3, 4, 5, 6, and 7). Then the communication plan is rolled out (corresponds to stage 8). Finally, follow-up with staff takes place at the end of the change process (corresponds to stage 9).

Galpin has identified a practical change management tool, which he calls a "cultural screen." This tool focuses on the cultural aspect of change and identifies those factors associated with the culture of the organization that should be assessed in order to achieve successful change. If, while using the screening tool, items are found that will impede the change process, a proactive approach to manage these specific items can be developed. If items are not identified prior to change efforts, then there is a risk that the change will be slow or arduous or will fail.

The cultural screening tool, which is used in implementing change (Galpin, 1996a), includes these nine items (see **Figure 4-5**):

- *Rules and policies*—To support positive implementation of change, identify and eliminate the rules and policies that will impede or "restrain" the change process. Develop new policies and procedures that will reinforce or "drive" the change. This corresponds to driving and restraining forces in Lewin's model.
- *Goals and measurement*—Develop clear goals and measurements that will reinforce the desired change. This will be needed for sustaining the change and holding the gains over time.
- *Customs and norms*—Replace the old way of doing things by making it harder to revert back and reinforce the new change by making it easier to implement.

Figure 4-5. Cultural Screening Tool

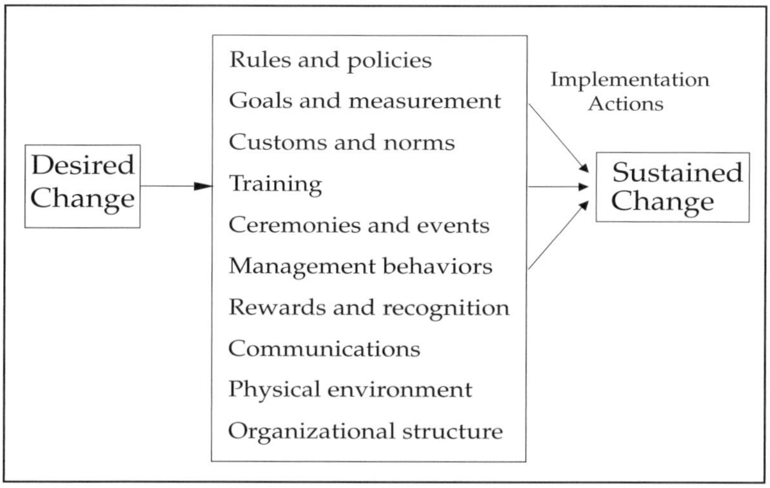

- *Training*—Develop training and education that will reinforce the new change. Provide real-time, hands-on experience with the new process to support acceptance.
- *Ceremonies and events*—Implement ceremonies that reinforce the new change and recognize both individual and team contributions to the success of the change effort.
- *Management behaviors*—Publicly recognize and reward managers who support and implement the change. Link pay, merit, and promotion to desired behaviors.
- *Rewards and recognition*—Make rewards specific to the change goals. Be sure that the performance system rewards the desired change. Rewards and recognition are key principles to successful management.
- *Communications*—Communicate in ways that demonstrate commitment to the change. Use multiple methods to deliver a consistent message throughout the change process.
- *Physical environment*—Ensure that the physical environment reflects and supports the change.
- *Organizational structure*—Ensure that the organizational structure reinforces the change (Galpin, 1996a).

In a humanistic approach to change, communication during all stages of the change process is critical for success. Communication should be realistic and honest, and it must be proactive, not reactive. Messages should be linked to the purpose of the change and should be repeated consistently through the entire process. Multiple avenues of communication are needed, including a feedback mechanism. This includes communication up and down as well as across the organization. Most experts on change reiterate that the most important aspect of change is communication, communication, communication.

Because communication is an essential aspect of Galpin's humanistic approach to change, it is important to discuss some associated pitfalls. Leaders must be clear and precise as to the change. If the leaders cannot succinctly and accurately describe the change, then inaccuracies and rumors will abound throughout the organization. Leaders who believe in limiting information will quickly find that the "grapevine" is a powerful force and that the desired message will not be delivered as intended. Open, honest communication is important to create credibility and trust. Leaders who are promoting significant change cannot delegate communication and ownership of the change to others. A well-written communication plan with senior leader involvement will be necessary throughout the entire change process. A common pitfall is to slow down communication once the process is under way. Ensuring that the change is completed and sustained is one of the more difficult tasks and often is overlooked or neglected. Leaders need to communicate with staff even after the change has been made to ensure it persists.

Management strategies based on Galpin's humanistic model focus specifically on assessing the organization's culture. This approach allows for the elimination of rules and policies that hinder the change and the development of new ones that reinforce the desired approach/behavior (similar to driving and restraining forces). These strategies also should include the development of goals and measurements that reinforce the desired changes. This provides greater leverage for advancing change.

E. Kotter's Heart of Change Model

John Kotter has written extensively on leadership and change management. His view on change is based on ensuring that people fully accept and incorporate the change into their belief system. His work also details a humanistic approach to get to the "heart" or emotional/feeling aspects associated with change (Kotter & Cohen, 2002). Kotter describes an eight-step model and cites numerous examples to help leaders manage change.

Step 1. Increase urgency. The first and most critical step in Kotter's model is to shake up the status quo and create a feeling of urgency. At this stage, people must be shocked into action ("We must do something!") The major challenge at this stage is to get people ready to move. Methods that will advance this stage include dramatic presentations with compelling stories and items that people can actually see, touch, and feel such as seeing a visual display of performance levels, touching a new computer, or feeling the emotional fear of job reductions. This step requires evidence that change is actually required.

Step 2. Build the guiding team. The next step is to organize a team of influential, effective leaders. It is important to get the right people in the right place with the right change process. They must be fully committed to the change initiative, be well-respected within the organization, and have power and influence to drive the change effort. It is a challenge to get the right people with the tools to be an effective trusted team. The team makeup should be diverse enough to provide multiple perspectives of the change and the stakeholders' interests.

Step 3. Get the vision right. As with other models presented, a clear vision is essential. Without clear directions the team cannot focus on the change and the implementation process. Providing this direction is leadership's responsibility. It is the vision that will steer the team into the new direction. Visioning activities about possible futures will help create strategies for the change initiative.

Step 4. Communicate for buy-in. It has already been said: communicate, communicate, communicate! Once a vision and strategy have been developed, they must be communicated to the organization. Sending clear, credible, and heartfelt messages about the direction of change establishes genuine, gut-level buy-in, which sets the stage for getting people to act. Keep communication simple and sincere; find out what people are really feeling and address their anxiety, confusion, anger, and distrust. Rid communication channels of "junk" so that the important message can be delivered. This step should be constantly reassessed throughout the change effort.

Step 5. Empower action. The next step is to empower people to take action by removing barriers. Removing obstacles will promote confidence in change, allowing more people to feel able to act.

Step 6. Create short-term wins. Short-term wins provide visible immediate successes and inspire people to believe that the change can be implemented. The challenge is to create short-term wins and energize users of the change.

Step 7. Don't let up. The process is not complete until the change is a reality. Leaders need to support the change over time, building on the momentum of short-term wins by keeping the sense of urgency alive. It is difficult to sustain excitement and energy over time and easy to become sidetracked by other tasks.

Step 8. Make change stick. The end of the change process often is one of the most difficult stages. Once the change is implemented, it must be ingrained in the organization, so that gains can be sustained, and a return to the previous way of doing things is prevented (Kotter & Cohen, 2002).

F. Prochaska's Transtheoretical Change Model

James Prochaska's approach to changing behavior is known as the transtheoretical, or "stages of change," model (Prochaska & DiClemente, 1999). The concepts of this model have been applied to numerous individual behaviors, including those related to maintaining a healthy weight and smoking cessation. The stages of change explain the individual's readiness to change behavior, rather than a process change. This model is useful for working with individual staff, patients, and providers to change behaviors.

Six stages that individuals use to change behavior (based on psychotherapy) are identified, including

- *Precontemplation*—there is no intention to take action within the next 6 months
- *Contemplation*—there is an intention to take action within the next 6 months
- *Preparation*—there is an intention to take action within the next 30 days and there have been some behavioral steps in this direction
- *Action*—behavior has changed for less than 6 months
- *Maintenance*—behavior has changed for more than 6 months
- *Termination*—the behavior will never return and there is complete confidence in the ability to cope without fear of relapse (Prochaska & DiClemente, 1999).

Figure 4-6 illustrates the sequence of changes along a time continuum. Prochaska, Director of the Cancer Prevention Research Center (CPRC), has led the development of measures that can be used with the Transtheoretical Model. All assessment inventories are available for research purposes only and are not for clinical use (http://www.uri.edu/research/cprc/measures.htm). Measures

Figure 4-6. Stages in Changing Behavior

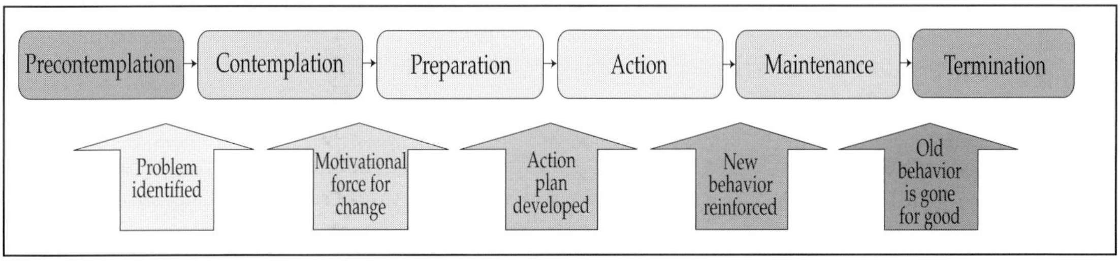

are available on the following topics: smoking, alcohol, cocaine, mammography, exercise, sun protection, coping and stress, weight control, psychotherapy, HIV and safer sex, and substance abuse.

Using this model requires some different strategies than the previous models presented. This model assumes that a person will not change his or her behavior until ready. Therefore, planned change is dependent on the readiness of the individual, not the organization. The person must move from a state of precontemplation to contemplation; only when this has occurred can change actually take place. The application of this model may be useful with special populations and health behavior changes, such as congestive heart failure patients and smoking cessation, adherence to medication regimen, and weight-loss programs. It also may be effective with individual provider practice patterns, for example, influencing providers to adopt a new product or technology. It will not be as useful for planned system change.

G. Change Models Summary

Six change models have been presented to help in understanding different ways to think about change and how various strategies, techniques, or tools can be used to effect change based on these models. This list is not meant to be exhaustive, but rather to provide a working knowledge about change and common strategies. No single model will fit every type of change or organization. For this reason, healthcare quality professionals need a repertoire of skills or a toolkit from which to draw for each situation.

Models explain a particular phenomenon and provide a view so techniques can be applied at strategic points. There are many common elements or similarities among the models, such as movement from a current state to a future state (see Figure 4-1). The impetus for this transition is dissatisfaction with the current state. Some common elements among models include readiness for change, communication of the change, and leadership for implementing the change. Using an approach in which change is planned provides the best results for a successful change.

Similarities in models also include the characteristics of the change itself and how these characteristics make it more likely or less likely to be readily accepted by users. Common factors are also identified in each model that will increase the speed of change within an organizational setting. The primary differences in the models are the scope and level of change. Most of the models address complex changes within organizations that often involve systems and processes; Prochaska's model focuses on individual behavior changes.

III. Change Management

Planning and managing change will be described in three major areas including the assessment of readiness for change, plan-do-study-act (PDSA) cycles of change, and change concepts.

A. Assessing Readiness for Change

Several tools have been described to assist in assessing an organization or unit for change. This first step is critical if the change is to be successful. If the organization is not ready or has many forces that will prove to be obstacles, then it is likely that the change may be slow or may not succeed at all. It is this human side of change that is critical to manage. If the assessment demonstrates a high degree of readiness, then the next steps of the change process can proceed.

It is important to reiterate that "All changes do not necessarily lead to improvement, but all improvement requires change" (IHI, "How to Improve" [n.d., paragraph 6]). This concept has been strongly voiced by the IHI, which also provides several tools for performance improvement that will now be addressed.

The point of change is to make an improvement. Until now the discussion has focused on change models; it now moves to a performance improvement model to make change for improvement. There are variations to the original PDCA model, including plan-do-study-act (PDSA; see **Figure 4-7**), FOCUS-PDCA, and others. The basic PDSA model is used to further explain change management, but remember that no single model or approach will fit every need. The approach must be tailored to each organization.

Figure 4-7. Process Improvement Model (PDSA)

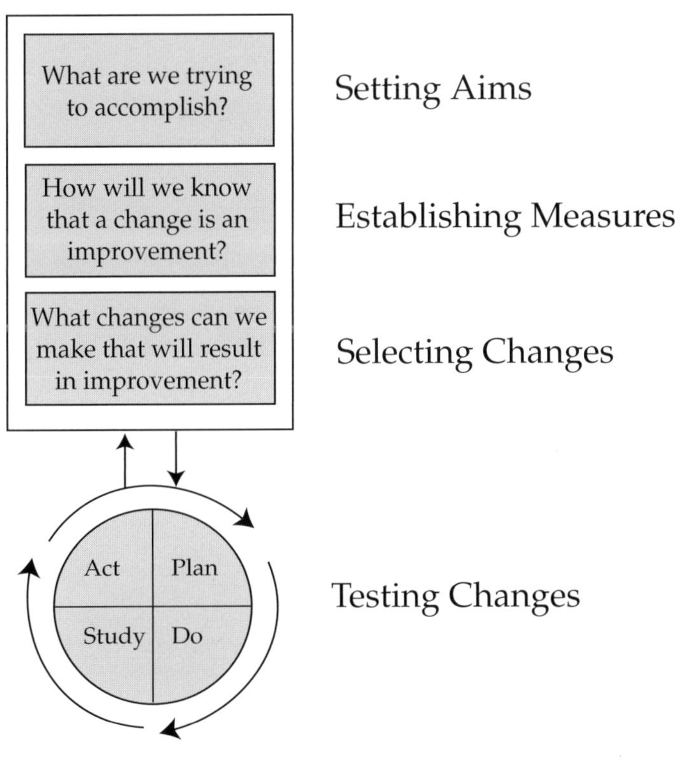

Reprinted from www.IHI.org with permission of the Institute for Healthcare Improvement. ©2004.

Figure 4-8 illustrates in a simple manner how to assess readiness for change. If the organization is ready and a plan is followed, chances for success are good. If the organization is not ready, the change agent must determine whether she or he can help to make the organization ready or whether the change should instead be considered at a later time. If a change effort proceeds in an organization that is not ready, the costs of failure will be high.

Other tools can be found in Module One, Foundation, Techniques, and Tools.

Figure 4-8. Assessing Readiness for Change

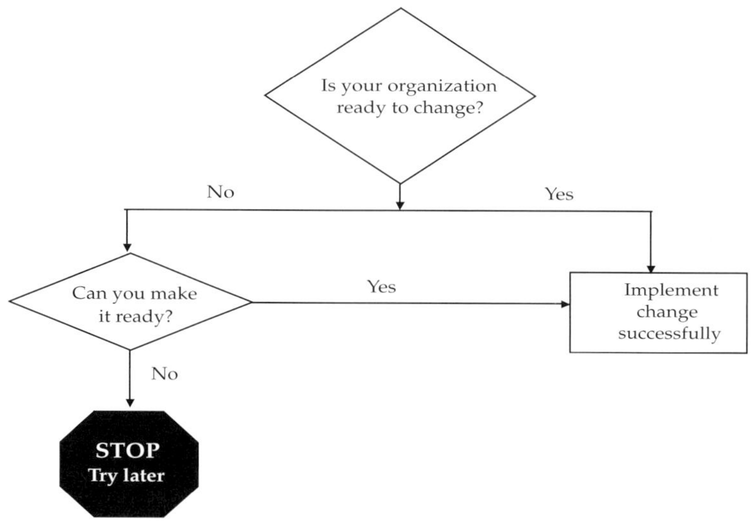

Reprinted with permission from Making change work: Practical tools for overcoming human resistance to change *by Brien Palmer. © 2004, ASQ Quality Press, Milwaukee, WI.*

B. PDSA Cycles of Change

Specific strategies that can be used to test and link tests of change using PDSA cycles and the IHI model (IHI, *Linking Tests of Change* [n.d.]; *Tips for Testing Changes* [n.d.]) include the following:

- Plan for multiple cycles of improvement in advance to support rapid cycle movement.
- Scale the scope and size of tests so that small tests can be done rapidly (e.g., with a few patients, one provider, or in a single day).
- Choose people who want to work on the improvement change process.
- Capitalize on existing resources, best practice, and research. Don't reinvent the wheel.
- Select "easy, visible wins" or "low-hanging fruit" changes first. Make the test feasible and practical.
- Don't delay a project because technology is not available; for small projects, paper and pen or other simple methods may be sufficient.
- Collect useful, meaningful measures and review results of every change cycle to determine any modifications that are needed.
- Test the change under a variety of conditions (e.g., different shifts and weekends).
- Be prepared to stop or abandon the process if there is no improvement.

C. Change Concepts

Langley, Nolan, Nolan, Norman, and Provost (1996) introduced the idea of *change concept* as a general approach to develop specific ideas for improvement. Nine change concepts have been identified; these can be further subdivided into 70 major ideas. The nine primary change concepts, which fit the PDSA improvement cycle, have been identified as ways to introduce creative or innovative approaches to change and improvement. They are as follows:

- Eliminate waste.
- Improve work flow.
- Optimize inventory.
- Change the work environment.
- Enhance producer/customer interface.
- Manage time.
- Manage variation.
- Design error-proof systems.
- Focus on the product or service.

IV. Factors That Affect Change

A. Factors That Support Successful/Accelerated Change

A number of factors have been identified as accelerators for success. There are several different ways to think about these factors. For example, change is accelerated when the organization has a culture that encourages and has a capacity for continuous learning. Having knowledge of its customers and key business processes will allow an organization to identify driving and restraining forces quickly and move into the phases of planned change more easily. Every change requires some access to resources. The availability of resources such as training, project materials, information systems, personnel, and financial support will accelerate the change process. **Table 4-3** summarizes different aspects of an organization and those characteristics that accelerate change and innovation.

In addition, these characteristics and values of high-performing organizations have been identified in the *2005 Baldrige Health Care Criteria for Perfomance Excellence* (Baldrige National Quality Program, 2005):

- Leadership systems are designed to achieve results (strong leadership).
- Strategy is generally simple and aligned with operations and deployed at all levels.
- Design and maintenance of the organizational culture is an intentional act of leadership.
- There is a clear understanding of the mission and vision at all levels of the organization with a focus on the future (visionary).
- "Rapid response" is employed.
- Desired results are defined, measured, and aligned with strategy, thereby creating value (results-driven).
- Decisions are based on sound data (manage by facts).
- Customer focus is a foundation of the culture, with patient-focused excellence.
- Measurement is deployed at all levels and owned by those doing the work (demand quality throughout).
- Innovation is valued and encouraged.
- Partnerships and alliances that value staff and partners are created.
- Continuous improvement and process management are integrated into daily work (seek continuous improvement).
- Organizational and personal learning are valued and integrated into work process.
- Human resource practices are designed to support the desired organizational culture.
- Employees are involved and there is focus on people and systems. Work is performed by teams. Decision making is done at the lowest level possible.

Table 4-3. High-Performing Organizations: Factors That Affect Speed of Change

Aspect of Organization	Accelerator of Change/Innovation
Leadership	• is active, visible, and supportive of change. • makes change focus/goal clear. • is strong communicator of the change. • is accountable for the change (ownership and not delegation). • involves all leaders. • expects results. • manages perceptions and expectations.
Culture	• assesses readiness for the change. • supports creativity, innovation, and risk-taking. • accepts failures (without blame), as well as successes. • encourages new ideas. • supports participative structure with staff level involvement. • focuses on group learning. • values continuous learning and improvement. • encourages diversity. • focuses on systems and processes. • rewards individuals and teams for performance. • values relationships.
Structure	• develops strong team infrastructure with empowerment. • makes resources available for the change.
Techniques	• make tools available to teams. • use available tools and technology. • apply change models and concepts. • use constraints and forcing functions. • replace old ways of doing things with new customs/norms and reinforce the change. • use training that reinforces the change. • put procedures in place to reinforce the change. • recognize and reward by linking promotion and pay to desired behaviors. • make it easy to accomplish the change. • simplify, standardize, and use technology wisely.

Sources: Baldrige National Quality Program, 2005; Fraser & Schall, 2002.

- Focus is on improving employee knowledge and skill.
- Social responsibility and attention to the health of the community is integrated into the organization.
- Systems perspective is an organizational characteristic.

Organizations exhibiting these characteristics and values have a greater capacity to adapt to change and to implement more innovations than organizations that do not.

B. Factors That Reduce Resistance to Change

In managing resistance to change, three key areas need to be assessed: attitude, skill, and knowledge. Remember that fear accompanies change, and fear cannot be eliminated, so the change strategy needs to actively address this emotion. Fear is usually associated with the unknown effects that the change will bring. This fear can be reduced by clearly identifying the effect of the change effort and communicating openly with those involved.

- Strategies to reduce resistance in people who are not willing to make the change include setting goals, measuring performance, providing coaching and feedback, and rewarding and recognizing positive efforts.

- Strategies to reduce resistance in people who are not able to perform the new change include educating and training staff in the new skills and the use of various management techniques.
- Strategies to reduce resistance in people who do not have the necessary knowledge to make the change include
  - communicating the what, why, how, when, and who of the change process
  - presenting a positive outlook of the proposed change
  - having a clear focus and goal for the change and expectations of those involved
  - being flexible and adaptable during the change process
  - using a structured approach to manage ambiguity and confusion
  - planning and coordinating the change process in a systematic way with clear expectations
  - using a proactive rather than a reactive approach.

V. Innovation and Creativity

A. Creativity

If an organization desires a culture that is creative, resilient, regenerative, and that promotes learning, then it must look at human relationships. In this context, people are more willing to change and are more adaptable because they believe they are not alone and that together they can manage almost anything (this corresponds to individual resiliency and capacity to change).

To encourage creativity in an organization, leaders must be accessible and acknowledge the value of people's contributions. They must create opportunities in which people can take risks and be allowed to fail. Creativity is needed in organizations to generate new ideas, remain competitive, and face the constant barrage of new challenges. Hundreds of ideas must be generated to actually find a true innovation that can be implemented into practice (Plsek, 1996). Common themes of models of creativity now include

- Creative process involves purposeful, imaginative-idea-generation and critical evaluation.
- Purposeful generation of new ideas can be directed.
- The creative process requires action and implementation of ideas.

A number of techniques can be used to create new ideas:

- Break routine ways of thinking and conduct activities to generate ideas.
- Inspire breakthrough performance.
- Use brainstorming (and variations such as brainwriting).
- Use metaphors.
- Observe common activities and products.
- Look to other industries and disciplines for ideas.
- Use technology in new ways.
- Develop prototypes and models.
- Develop an idealized design.
- Use traditional tools such as fishbone (cause-and-effect or Ishikawa) diagrams, flowcharts, and process maps.
- List alternative uses for common products.

According to Plsek (1996), there are four general phases, or steps, of directed creativity:

1. preparation
   - pausing and noticing
   - seeking other points of view
   - refocusing a topic
   - looking closer and analyzing
   - searching for analogies
   - creating new worlds
2. imagination
   - brainstorming
   - using analogies
   - provoking imaginations
   - "leaping"
   - combining concepts systematically
   - organizing and displaying ideas
   - harvesting ideas
3. development
   - final harvesting
4. action.

These four phases include a structured approach within each phase to guide creativity and the generation of tangible ideas and/or products. Each phase can be enhanced with specific tools (**Figure 4-9**).

Figure 4-9. Four Phases of Directed Creativity

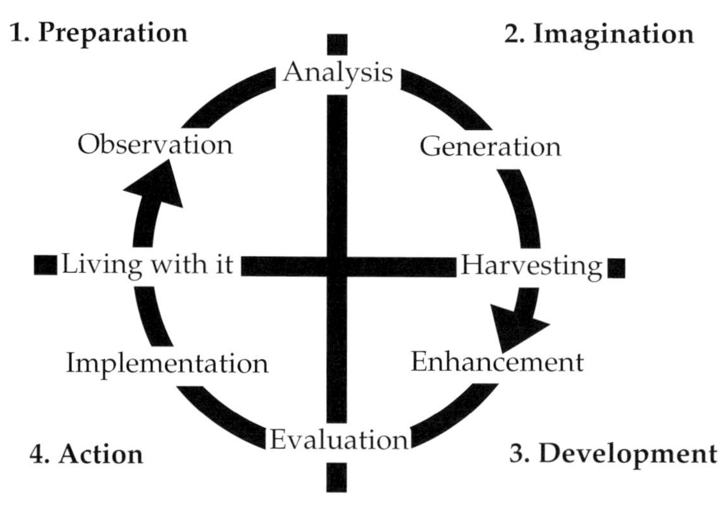

Reprinted with permission from Directed creativity cycle *published on http://www.directedcreativity.com/pages/CycleFrameset.html by Paul E. Plsek & Associates, Inc. © 1996.*

Although everyone has the capacity for creativity, it must be nurtured and identified as an expectation within the organizational culture. The three basic principles that underpin creative thinking are attention, escape, and movement. Plsek (1996) describes these principles—to focus attention, escape the current reality, and continue mental movement toward invention or generation of new ideas. The principle of attention primarily occurs in the preparation stage of creativity in which attention is focused on an idea or item in a different uncommon way. In order to see familiar objects in a new light, the principle of escape is used. By this Plsek (1996) means to escape the tendency to "oversimplify the world into neat conventional explanations." The principle of escape allows one to see old things in a new light. The third principle of movement is to move away from familiar or traditional ideas to an innovative or novel approach.

Bisognano and Plsek (2004) have also identified seven dimensions of the culture that promote creative thinking and the development of innovation. These seven dimensions are

1. Risk taking
2. Specific targets
3. Resources
4. Widely shared information
5. Tools and methods
6. Rewards
7. Relationships and teams.

Another model for creativity, called the "seven S model," describes successful characteristics for organizations, which must be aligned in order for creativity to be fostered (Higgins, 1995).

- *Strategy*—major set of plans through which an organization achieves its purpose while responding to and proactively changing its environment
- *Structure*—jobs, authority to do those jobs, departmentalization of jobs, and the manager's span of control
- *Systems*—processes and flows that allow an organization to get things done from day to day
- *Style*—consistent pattern of behavior when relating to staff and employees
- *Staff*—number and type of employees needed to perform the jobs
- *Shared values*—values understood and shared by all employees of an organization that make it unique
- *Skills*—capabilities that are possessed by the organization as a whole, as opposed to individual skills.

Once an organization has aligned the seven characteristics so that creativity is nurtured in the culture, innovations can emerge. There are some guidelines that can then help in transforming creative endeavors into innovations. These nine rules of innovation can be adopted by the organization as strategies:

- Innovate or imitate best-performing innovative organizations.
- Practice both research and development and search and development. Do not reinvent the wheel.
- Engage in both product and process innovation. Most healthcare organizations implement process innovations.
- Invest in new processes and products as well as in old ones. Each product and process has a typical life span and these products and processes should be maximized during this period.
- Practice both "big bang" (breakthrough) innovation and continuous (incremental) improvement.
- Be both market- and technology-driven.
- Be totally committed to innovation as a strategy.
- Conduct both basic and applied research in a coordinated way and make basic research more applications-oriented.
- Use speed strategies to bring products to market.

Creativity and innovation can be thought of as "Yin and Yang." Each is essential to the other and to successful organizations. Creativity is necessary for innovations and innovations depend on a creative organization (**Figure 4-10**).

Figure 4-10. Interdependence of Creativity and Innovation

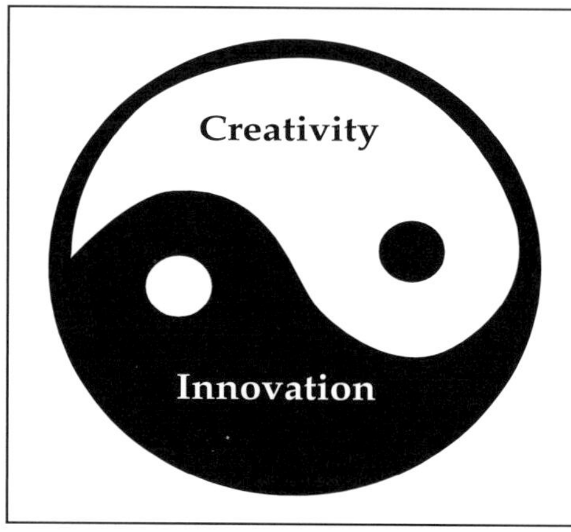

In the *2005 Baldrige Health Care Criteria for Performance Excellence* (Baldrige National Quality Program, 2005), there is a focus on managing for innovation, defined as "making meaningful change to improve an organization's services, processes and operations to create new value for the organization's stakeholders" (p. 3). Managing for innovation should lead to new dimensions of performance. Innovation builds on the knowledge of the organization and its staff. This core concept is found in Strategic Planning, Category 2.1, on strategy development; Measurement, Analysis, and Knowledge Management, Category 4.1, on measurement, analysis, and review of organizational performance; and Staff Focus, Category 5.1, on work systems.

B. Complexity Theory

Because complexity science and theory is an emerging field and has only recently been applied to healthcare, it has not traditionally been presented in literature on change management. However, many of the principles of complex systems provide an explanation for certain aspects of organizational behaviors, such as the importance of relationships, unpredictability of evolution, size of outcomes not related to size of inputs, and the interdependence of elements in a system. Understanding the complexity of the healthcare system can help change agents in using different strategies to influence change.

Complexity theory can explain how simple principles found in nature (e.g., how birds flock) apply to complex human organizations. Several rules guide natural phenomena and exhibit underlying patterns or intrinsic order. Complexity theory is based on a systems approach and uses a few simple rules to guide the interaction between the components of a system. The rules include the following principles:

- Managers should focus on relationships at all levels within their organizations.
- Small changes can have large effects.
- Interesting and unpredictable properties can be expected to emerge from a system.

Complexity theory underscores the importance of relationships. How people relate to one another affects what emerges in the organization—the culture, the creativity, the productivity. Understanding and modifying culture is a key to successful change strategies; changes often fail when the impact of culture is neglected or minimized. Cultural change is closely tied to individual change, so many of the change concepts discussed earlier may come into play.

The important notion in complexity theory is not the size, but rather the impact of the change. Small changes can have a large impact. It is for this reason that complexity theory is included in this section on change management. By understanding some different theoretical perspectives, it is possible to approach organizational change in new and different ways. This theoretical framework requires a major shift in thinking. If small changes can have a large impact, then the change agent must be able to discern which changes to implement and how to allow the natural order to prevail.

Complex systems have three primary zones of functioning (Plsek, 1996; Zimmerman, Lindberg, & Plsek, 2001):

- stable zone (stagnant state without growth or change)
- chaotic zone (haphazard state with constant crises, little productivity, and great stress)
- creative zone (state of expected fluctuation, which creates the necessary tension for new ideas to be generated).

VI. Spread of Change and Innovation: Rogers' Diffusion Model

To be widely implemented, new ideas, products, or technology must be disseminated throughout an organization. *Diffusion* is the process by which an innovation or new idea is communicated through certain channels over time among members of a social system (*dissemination* is synonymous with diffusion for purposes of this work). An *innovation* is an idea, practice, or object that is perceived as new by those who adopt it. The directed creativity activities may lead to an innovation or the innovation may be adopted from the outside.

The main elements of Rogers' (1995) diffusion model include

- innovation
- communication channels about the innovation
- time (time span from the point of first hearing of the innovation to the point of decision to accept or reject it, the number of individuals in a social system who adopt an innovation in a given period, and the innovativeness of the individual or agency that determines the time needed to achieve adoption)
- social system in which an innovation is adopted.

The innovation-decision process consists of five stages. Before the five stages occur, however, other factors must be considered. These prior conditions include

- previous practice (history and culture of change in the organization and support by leaders)
- needs of the organization within a competitive market
- innovativeness of the organization
- norms of the system (culture of change, readiness for change, boundaries and relationships, channels of communication, and priorities of the organization).

Rogers (1995) defines five stages in adopting an innovation, as follows:

1. Knowledge (socioeconomic characteristics, personality variables, communication behavior); the level of the person's innovativeness determines the type of adopter
2. Persuasion (perceived characteristics of the innovation: relative advantage, compatibility, complexity, trialability, or suitability for trial, observability-visibility, reversibility, uncertainty)
3. Decision (adoption/rejection)
4. Implementation (direct application, reinvention, indirect application/effect)
5. Confirmation (evaluation of the innovation's effectiveness to determine its continuance or discontinuance).

According to Rogers (1995) the dissemination or diffusion of innovations is focused on influence in the following three major areas. This model was adapted to healthcare by Berwick (2003).

- Perceptions of the innovation
  - — perceived benefit of the change/innovation (people are more likely to adopt a change/innovation if they think it can help them)
  - — compatibility of the change/innovation with the values, beliefs, past history, and current needs of individuals (people are more likely to adopt a change/innovation that is consistent with their own values)
  - — complexity of the change/innovation (as a general rule, simple changes/innovations are adopted faster than complicated ones)
  - — trialability of the change/innovation by users (people are more likely to adopt a change/innovation that they can try before being required to use it)
  - — observability of the change/innovation by people who can watch others try the change first (people are more likely to adopt a change/innovation that they can see in use before they have to actually use it).
- Characteristics of individuals who may (or may not) adopt the change, based on their degree of innovativeness
  - — innovators (2.5%)
  - — early adopters (13.5%)
  - — early majority (34%)
  - — late majority (34%)
  - — laggards (16%)
- Managerial and contextual factors within organizations involving communication, incentives, leadership, and management. The rate of adoption of innovations is greater with increased communication, positive incentives, and supportive leaders.

By using the information from Rogers' model, healthcare quality professionals can develop plans that incorporate these concepts, increasing the likelihood that the change/innovation will be successfully implemented.

The percentage of individuals within specific adopter categories matches the bell curve shown in **Figure 4-11.** The rate of adoption of specific innovations can be affected by strategies to target specific adopter groups. Targeting innovators and early adopters is usually sufficient to create the necessary support and momentum for adoption of change/innovation, with the other groups following (Rogers, 1995).

Tools also have been developed to assess the rate of adoption of innovations. The scorecard tool (**Table 4-4**) can be used to assess the possibility for and rate of adoption of an innovation or new change based on specific criteria defined in Rogers' model (IHI, "Tips for Testing Change" [n.d.]). If the assessment indicates that the adoption is not likely to be successful, additional strategies can be developed to improve the odds.

Figure 4-11. Adopter Categories for Innovations

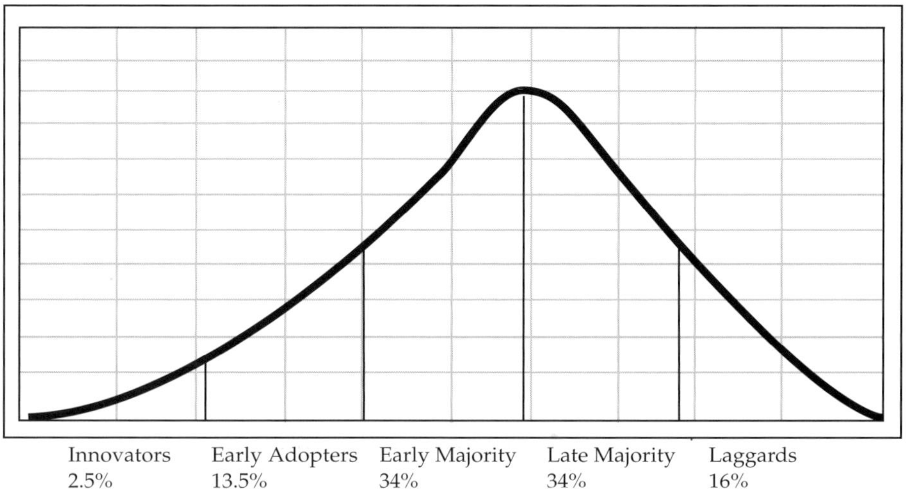

The higher the rating of each item on the scorecard, the greater the likelihood that a specific innovation and/or change will be successfully adopted. The items in the scorecard are defined as follows:

- *Relative advantage*—the degree to which an innovation is perceived as better than the idea it supersedes
- *Simplicity/complexity*—the degree to which an innovation is perceived as simple to understand and use
- *Compatibility*—the degree to which an innovation is perceived as being consistent with the existing values, experiences, beliefs, and needs of potential adopters
- *Trialability, or suitability for trial*—the degree to which an innovation can be tested on a small scale
- *Observability/visibility*—the degree to which the use of an innovation and the results it produces are visible to those who should consider it
- *Communicability*—the ability to clearly communicate a description and value of the innovation to stakeholders
- *Reversibility*—the ability to stop the adoption or use of the innovation and return to a normal or "safe" position if the innovation is not effective
- *Uncertainty*—the fear and discomfort associated with the implementation of the innovation (IHI, [n.d.]).

This aspect of dissemination or diffusion has been addressed by the IHI with a model for spreading change and innovations to promote rapid dissemination of

Table 4-4. New Idea Scorecard Tool

	Relative Advantage	Simplicity	Compatibility	Trialability or Suitability for Trial	Observability
______ name of innovation	______ score	______ score	______ score	______ score	______ score

quality improvement practices across an organization. This framework (**Figure 4-12**) includes seven major components to be considered broadly and not in a specific order (IHI, "Spreading Change" [n.d.]).

Figure 4-12. A Framework for Spread

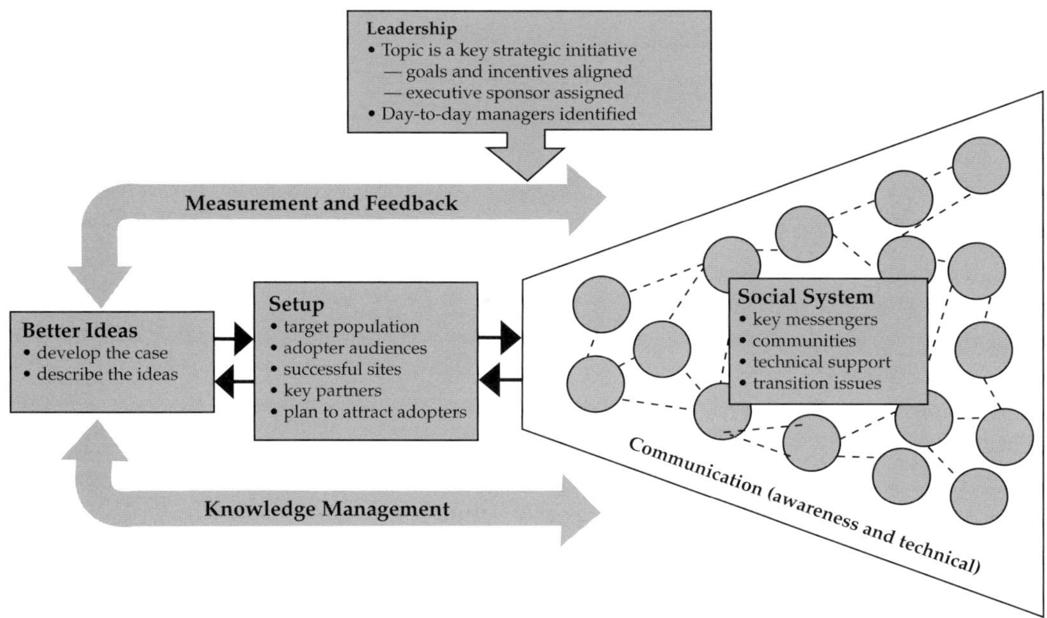

Reprinted from www.IHI.org with permission of the Institute for Healthcare Improvement. © 2004.

The elements of the spread framework are as follows:

- *Leadership*—Leadership is required to ensure that the goal to be spread throughout the organization is aligned with strategic goals. Responsibility for day-to-day leadership must be assigned to provide guidance on the spread. Communication channels need to be established and supported by leaders as part of an ongoing process.
- *Setup for spread (infrastructure)*—This component describes a structure to coordinate the activities in which the target population is identified, the sites selected for initiating the spread, key partners, and a plan for implementation.
- *Better ideas*—This refers to the changes or improvement ideas that have been demonstrated as successful and are desired to be spread throughout the organization.
- *Communication*—Communication is a key underpinning of the spread model, in which strategies include the purpose and methods of communication for the target population.
- *Social system*—The social system for spread includes the individuals and groups in the target population. The social system relationships must be understood so that communication, support, and issues can be identified and resolved.
- *Knowledge management*—Knowledge management is the process of collecting information about the spread with the measurement and feedback component

for modifying the spread process as necessary. Knowledge management focuses on the knowledge that people need to do their work, improve services, remain current with changing needs, and develop innovative solutions (Baldrige National Quality Program, 2005). Knowledge management is the process through which organizations actually create value from knowledge-based assets. Most often, generating value from these assets involves sharing in an effort to devise best practices. Not all information is valuable, so it is up to individual organizations to determine what information qualifies as knowledge-based assets. The challenge inherent with knowledge is figuring out how to recognize, generate, share, and manage it to foster innovations.

- *Measurement and feedback*—A system for measurement and feedback is needed to ensure the spread of the change proceeds as planned. This system provides data about the process and outcomes. In combination with knowledge management, these components allow adjustments in the spread strategy.

To maximize results, a strategy is needed to spread change/improvements. These strategies include assessing readiness for spread, developing the plan, leveraging pilot sites, developing a communication plan, and developing a measurement and feedback system.

Communication methods for spreading change are important. The range of communication methods and the associated purpose are shown in **Figure 4-13**.

Figure 4-13. The Range of Communication Methods

Purpose

Share Information ←——————————→ Shape Behavior

Communication Methods

General publications	Personal touch	Interactive activities	Public events	Face-to-face sharing

VII. Special Populations and Considerations

A. Special Patient Populations

A major portion of the discussion thus far has been on organizational change or process change, primarily affecting employees within an organization. An area that also must be considered in terms of change management is special populations. Both individual and patient populations often require behavioral changes in healthcare practices. The change management approaches commonly are needed for patients with chronic conditions such as congestive heart failure, renal failure, or diabetes. Other patients who have complex medication or treatment schedules also may require change management. Some examples in which individual or patient groups require change management include

- substance abuse and behavioral changes necessary to quit using (e.g., tobacco, alcohol, and illegal substances)
- dietary and weight management (e.g., bowel disorders, obesity, eating disorders, and diabetes)
- mental health disorders (e.g., medication compliance and therapeutic behaviors).

B. Providers

Change management techniques also are utilized with specific providers, such as physicians, to engage them as champions of a change initiative or to enlist them in making a major change. For example, providers must play a leadership role in implementation of computerized physician order entry (CPOE), yet also are key users in actually implementing the change to CPOE. Physician providers can offer unique barriers and resistance to change. Many change efforts affecting physicians require standardization (e.g., those related to surgical supplies and clinical guidelines). Physicians often term this standardized approach as "cookbook medicine" and resist it as being an intrusion into their practice. Change strategies require special attention to these restraining forces and to the development of culture and methods to communicate rationale for the change. Driving forces for this group often include a demonstration of the investment or incentive to change, such as the relevance to practice or pay for performance. The last change factor to consider with this group is accountability and how it can be applied in implementing and evaluating the change. The desire to apply best practices or evidence-based practice often is a strong driving force for change with this particular group.

VIII. Role of Research

Research plays a key role in implementing change in the practice setting. Two models that can help put research into practice are presented.

A. Havelock's Change Agent Model

Ronald Havelock (1973) added additional concepts to the knowledge of utilization theory by proposing the "linker" system to transfer new knowledge, skills, or products. This model describes the link between the user system and a change agent. The change process involves six steps:

- need
- problem diagnosis
- search for resources
- retrieval of information/ideas
- development of a solution
- application.

In Havelock's model a special change agent, who is usually external to an organization, is needed to help the organization implement research findings and make changes necessary to implement a new practice (Havelock, 1973).

B. Stetler's Research Utilization Model

A model for research utilization in nursing was developed in 1976 and advanced by Stetler in 1994 (Stetler, 1994; 2001). This framework utilizes many of the change concepts to apply and evaluate research for utilization in practice. The steps in the model are as follows.

Step 1. Preparation. The first phase involves determination of the purpose and the focus of the research review. The literature is widely reviewed for studies on topics or practices that an organization wants to evaluate to meet a specific need. The purpose may be to solve a problem; provide the basis for a policy, standard, or protocol; or prepare for an educational program.

Step 2. Validation. In this phase, research reports are critiqued by members of the organization for scientific merit. Decisions are made as to whether the findings are useful to the organization or individual conducting the utilization project. At this point a decision is made either to move to Step 3 or not to proceed.

Step 3. Comparative evaluation. There are four parts to this phase, in which a meta-analysis is conducted to compare different studies on a particular topic. The steps are

- substantiating evidence
- determining the fit of the research to the organizational setting
- identifying the feasibility, risks, resources, and readiness to move forward with utilizing a particular research practice
- determining the current practice change that will need to be made.

Step 4. Decision making. Four types of decisions are now possible for an organization to make as to using the research in practice:

- to use the findings
- to consider using the findings
- to delay using the findings
- to not use the findings.

Step 5. Translation/application. This phase involves planning the actual implementation of the findings in practice, assuming that in Step 4 the organization decided to use the findings. This phase comprises the following steps for change:

- assess the situation to be changed
- develop a plan for change
- implement the plan.

Step 6. Evaluation. The final phase is to evaluate the impact of the research-based change on the organization (Stetler, 1994; 2001).

IX. Summary

A variety of change models with specific techniques has been presented. In addition, a discussion on innovation and creativity with models for spread has been provided. Considerations of special populations have been presented to describe how change management can be incorporated into clinical practice. A research utilization model has been described to entwine change management models with research and implement changes for evidence-based practice. In almost every discussion, a movement is required from a current state to a future state; this may involve applying creativity and identifying an innovation for implementation or applying research into practice. Change management is integral to all these activities.

In summary, this module assists the healthcare quality professional by providing models, tools, and techniques. Materials for managing change include three major areas:

1. Preparing for change
    - Why do we need to change?
    - What is the present state like?
    - What is the future state like?
    - What is going to change?
    - What is not going to change?
    - Where are we most vulnerable in making this change work?
    - What will be the key success factors in the future state?
2. Beginning the change
    - What is our change strategy?
    - How do we best operationalize change?

- How do we best use our change levers?
- How do we position change as a challenge?
- How do we minimize the impact of losses by those most affected by change?

3. Cementing the change
    - Ensure using the change levers effectively.
    - Ensure that units are aligned with changes.
    - Ensure that all staff are involved.
    - Understand the purpose of the change.
    - Understand desired outcomes of the change.
    - Determine roles in planning and implementation.
    - Acquire new behaviors needed for the change.

Change levers and techniques to ensure a successful change that have been presented include

- clear understanding of the need for change
- quality leadership
- commitment of sponsors
- clear vision of future and strategy
- change structure
- education and training
- effective communication
- measurement systems
- alignment of infrastructure
- reward systems
- organizational structure aligned
- skill of change agents.

Finally, key principles for effective change that have been presented include

- Communicate, communicate, communicate.
- Continuous improvement is key to success.
- Keep trying until you get it right.
- Invest in quick wins and celebrate successes.
- Think outside the box creatively and innovate.
- Create ownership and involvement.
- Walk the talk.
- Hold people accountable.

The reader now has a variety of tools to manage change successfully at the individual and organizational level.

References

Accel-team. (2004). *Change management. Achieving goal congruence.* Retrieved April 18, 2005, from www.accel-team.com/techniques/goal_congruence.html

American Psychological Association. (2003). *The road to resilience: What is resilience?* Retrieved April 18, 2005, from http://www.apahelpcenter.org/featuredtopics/feature.php?id=6

Baldrige National Quality Program. (2005). *Health care criteria for performance excellence.* Retrieved July 8, 2005, from www.quality.hist.gov/healthcare_criteria.htm

Berwick, D.M. (2003). Disseminating innovations in health care. *The Journal of the American Medical Association, 289*(15), 1969–1975.

Bisognano, M., & Plsek, P. (2004 December). *Top ten improvement ideas from 2004: Emerging and promising approaches.* Presented at the 16th Annual National Forum by the Institute for Healthcare Improvement in Orlando, Florida.

DeWeaver, M., & Gillespie, L. (1997). *Real world project management*. New York: Quality Resources.

Fraser, S.W., & Schall, M. (2002, December). *Accelerating the spread of better practice*. Presented at the 14th Annual Institute for Healthcare Improvement Conference in Orlando, FL.

Galpin, T.J. (1996a). Connecting culture to organizational change. *HR Magazine, 41*(30), 84–89.

Galpin, T.J. (1996b). *The human side of change*. San Francisco: Jossey-Bass Publishers.

Higgins, J.M. (1995). *Innovate or evaporate*. Winter Park, FL: New Management Publishing Company, Inc.

Institute for Healthcare Improvement. (n.d.). *How to improve. Improvement methods*. Retrieved April 18, 2005, from http://www.ihi.org/IHI/Topics/Improvement/Improvement Methods/HowToImprove/

Institute for Healthcare Improvement. (n.d.). *Linking tests of change*. Retrieved April 18, 2005, from www.ihi.org/IHI/Topics/Improvement/ImprovementMethods/HowTo Improve/rampsofchange.htm

Institute for Healthcare Improvement. (n.d.). *Spreading change*. Retrieved April 18, 2005, from www.ihi.org/IHI/Topics/Improvement/SpreadingChanges/Changes/

Institute for Healthcare Improvement. (n.d.). *Tips for testing changes*. Retrieved April 18, 2005, from www.ihi.org/IHI/Topics/Improvement/ImprovementMethods/HowTo Improve/tipfortestingchanges.htm

Kotter, J.P., & Cohen, D.S. (2002). *The heart of change*. Boston: Harvard Business School Publishing.

Langley, G.L., Nolan, K.M., Nolan, T.W., Norman, C.L., & Provost, L.P. (1996). *The improvement guide: A practical approach to enhancing organizational performance*. San Francisco: Jossey-Bass Publishers.

Palmer, B. (2004a). *Making change work: Practical tools for overcoming human resistance to change*. Milwaukee, WI: ASQ Quality Press.

Palmer, B. (2004b). Overcoming resistance to change. *Quality Progress, 37*(4), 35–39.

Plsek, P. (2002, December). *Complexity, culture and large-systems change*. Presented at the 14th Annual Institute for Healthcare Improvement Conference in Orlando, Florida.

Plsek, P.E. (1996). *Working paper: Models for the creative process*. Retrieved April 18, 2005, from www.directedcreativity.com/pages/WPModels.html

Pomeroy, A. (2004). Cooking up innovation. *HR Magazine, 49*(11), 46–53.

Prochaska, J.O., & DiClemente, C. (1999). *Transtheoretical model/stages of change*. Retrieved July 15, 2004, from http://www.hsc.usf.edu/~kmbrown/Stages_of_Change_Overview.htm

Rogers, E. (1995). *The diffusion of innovations* (5th ed.). New York: Free Press.

Schein, E.H. (n.d.). *Kurt Lewin's change theory in the field and in the classroom: Notes toward a model of managed learning*. Retrieved April 18, 2005, from www.solonline.org/res/wp/10006.html

Smith, M.K. (2004). *Kurt Lewin: Groups, experiential learning and action research*. Retrieved April 18, 2005, from www.infed.org/thinkers/et-lewin.htm

Zimmerman, B., Lindberg, C., & Plsek, P. (2001). *Edgeware. Insights from complexity science for health care leaders*. Irving, TX: VHA Inc.

Suggested Reading

Alemi, F. (2003). System thinking in a personal context to improve eating behaviors. *Journal for Healthcare Quality, 25*(2), 20–25.

Barrere, C. (2002). Changing attitudes among nurses and physicians: A step toward collaboration. *Journal for Healthcare Quality, 24*(3), 9–16, 56.

BRINT.com—The BigTech Network. *Complex systems articles, papers, books & bibliographies*. Retrieved April 18, 2005, from www.brint.com/systems.htm

Brown, D.S. (2003). Lessons in redesigning a quality program across the continuum. *Journal for Healthcare Quality, 25*(1), 36–42, 50.

Brown, E.J. (2004). Innovative ideas seminars: A method for eliciting innovations and their effect on quality and cost. *Journal for Healthcare Quality, 26*(5), 39–45.

Caudron, S. (2004). Taking charge of change. *Business Finance Magazine*. Retrieved April 18, 2005, from www.businessfinancemag.com/magazine/archives/

Hulse, K., Edmundson, L., Carroll, R., & Scholl, R.W. (2004). Diversion of controlled substances: A catalyst for change. *Journal for Healthcare Quality, 26*(5), 6–11.

Modernisation Agency. (2002, July). *From skepticism to support: What are the influencing factors?* Summary Report No. 1. Research into Practice Programme. Retrieved April 18, 2005, from http://www.modern.nhs.uk/scripts/default.asp?site_id=54&id=14993

Modernisation Agency. (2002, September). *Sustainability and spread in the National Booking Programme*. Summary Report No. 2. Research into Practice Programme. Retrieved April 18, 2005, from http://www.modern.nhs.uk/scripts/default.asp?site_id=54&id=14993

Moen, R., & Taylor, J. (2001). *Generating ideas for innovation: Some methods*. Presented at the 14th Annual Institute for Healthcare Improvement Conference in Orlando, FL.

Nickols, F. (2004). *Change management 101: A primer*. Retrieved April 18, 2005, from http://home.att.net/~nickols/change.htm

Prochaska, J. (n.d.). *Cancer Prevention Research Center Measures*. Retrieved April 21, 2005, from http://www.uri.edu/research/cprc/measures.htm

Riches, A. (n.d.). *Culture—Are you dancing with the devil*? Retrieved April 18, 2005, from www.anneriches.com.au/devil.html

Robertson, M.L. (2002). Reducing length of stay through rapid clinical redesign. *Journal for Healthcare Quality, 24*(5), 26–31.

Schoemer, K.G. (2004). *The new reality. How to make change your competitive advantage*. Brownsburg, IN: Penguin Press.

Shimabukuro, T.T., Kramer, J., & McGuire, M. (2004). Development and implementation of a nurse-managed anticoagulation program. *Journal for Healthcare Quality, 26*(1), 4–13, 60.

Tichy, N. (1997, April/May). Bob Knowling's change manual. *Fast Company, 8*, 76–82. Retrieved April 18, 2005, from http://www.fastcompany.com/online/08/change2.html

GLOSSARY

Accreditation. An external "seal of approval." Usually a voluntary process; accreditation indicates that a facility or service has passed a standardized objective review process (usually an on-site survey) conducted by an impartial organization and that it meets guidelines or nationally/internationally recognized performance standards.

Act. Process to implement changes on a broad scale.

Activity Network Diagram. Tool also known as an arrow diagram, program evaluation and review technique (PERT), or a critical path method (CPM) chart. Through the use of the arrow diagram, a sequence of events is depicted. It is useful when several simultaneous paths must be coordinated.

Administrative Support Information System. Information system that aids day-to-day operations in healthcare organizations, including financial information systems, human resources information systems, and office automation systems.

Affinity Diagram. Organizes numerous ideas or issues into groupings based on their natural relationships within the groupings. Typically used to analyze or chart a process and to structure and organize issues to provide a new perspective.

Balanced Scorecard (BSC). An approach to performance management developed by Norton and Vaplan. The basic idea of the BSC is that performance measures should provide a comprehensive view of organizational performance and not be overly dependent on a few choice indicators. The BSC helps organizations better link long-term strategy with short-term activities.

Baldrige Award. A competitive award that is given to organizations demonstrating a commitment to quality excellence based on successfully meeting the Baldrige National Healthcare Criteria for Performance Excellence.

Benchmarking. The comparison of an organization's or an individual practitioner's results against a reference point. Ideally, the reference point is a demonstrated best practice.

Black Belt. Member of the organization who has been extensively trained in Six Sigma methods. A Black Belt also is experienced in statistical analysis and interested in teaching others.

Brainstorming. A free-flowing generation of ideas with the potential to create excitement, equalize involvement, and result in original solutions to the problem.

Brainwriting. Tool used to aid in sharing ideas in which people who have ideas can make them anonymously. Reduces sense that one has to compete with others to be heard and often results in generation of more ideas than brainstorming.

Budgeting. Formal annual or periodic process through which financial performance goals and actual results are evaluated for the current and previous fiscal years. This allows for the development of formal goals for the next fiscal year.

Capital Budgeting. The process by which an organization evaluates and selects which long-term investments (or capital expenditures) it will make. Typically this is an annual activity, but it also may be triggered by events such as requests for new programs or equipment.

Case Management. Approach to care that consists of intake and assessment, development of care plan, case coordination, discharge planning, and quality management.

Cause-and-Effect, Ishikawa, or Fishbone Diagram. Diagram used to analyze and display the potential causes of a problem or the source of variation. In general, there are at least four categories in the diagram such as the four Ms: manpower, methods, machines, and materials, or the five Ps: patron (users of the system), people (workers), provisions (supplies), places to work (work environment), and procedures (methods and rules).

Centers for Medicare & Medicaid Services (CMS). Federal government agency within the U.S. Department of Health and Human Services that is accountable for Medicare, Medicaid, and state Children's Health Improvement Programs (CHIPs); formerly the Health Care Financing Administration (HCFA).

Certified Professional in Healthcare Quality (CPHQ). Designation received after passing the written examination and adhering to standards established by the Healthcare Quality Certification Board (HQCB) and continuing to maintain those standards through the recertification process.

Check. Measured outcomes compared to predicted outcomes.

Chi-square (χ^2) Test. Measures the statistical significance of a difference in proportions and is the most commonly reported statistical test in the medical literature.

Clinical Information System. Designed to support direct patient care processes; automated clinical information systems have great potential for analyzing and improving the quality of patient care. Expanded clinical information systems in use include medical records and their retrieval systems, computer-assisted medical decision making for history and physicals and antibiotic selection, and clinical application programs for health risk programs and health maintenance organization encounter data.

Clinical Risk Management. Used to indicate the concern and interest taken in clinical care provided to patients, clients, and other customers.

Cluster Sampling. Method requires that the population be divided into groups or clusters.

Coaching. The consultative, collaborative interaction of at least two people, characterized by advocacy and encouragement.

Code-Based System. Information system based on retrospective administrative data, such as data in the Uniform Bill document 1992 (UB-92) or claims data, including clinical information spanning the patient's entire stay but not identifying the specific timing of certain conditions.

College of American Pathologists (CAP). In addition to general laboratory accreditation, CAP also provides specialty programs for reproductive laboratories and forensic urine drug testing programs.

Commission of Office Laboratory Accreditation (COLA). Accredits physician office laboratories in compliance with clinical laboratory improvement amendments (CLIAs), hospitals, and independent laboratories.

Commission on Accreditation of Rehabilitation Facilities (CARF). Accreditation commission that promotes the quality, value, and optimal outcomes of services through a consultative accreditation process.

Common Cause. In statistical process control (SPC), it describes problems rooted in basic processes and systems.

Communicability. The ability to clearly communicate a description and value of the innovation to stakeholders.

Compatibility. The degree to which an innovation is perceived as being consistent with the existing values, experiences, beliefs, and needs of potential adopters.

Complex Adaptive System (CAS). A system of interdependent things (e.g., agents that can be people, departments) wherein there are a great number of connections between a wide variety of elements in addition to the ability to learn from experience.

Complex Process. Process that has uncertain outcomes even when formulas or prescriptive procedures have been developed and expertise is available (e.g., successful staffing of a nursing unit for one next shift does not necessarily ensure the success of the next).

Compliance. Conformity in fulfilling official requirements.

Complicated Process. Process that requires a high level of expertise in many specialized fields and coordination to achieve a high degree of certainty of the outcome (e.g., launching a moon rocket where the formulas are critical and necessary, and one successful launch increases the likelihood that the next launch will occur as planned).

Confidence Interval (CI). Provides a range of possible values around a sample estimate (e.g., a mean, proportion, ratio) that is calculated from data; commonly is used when comparing groups but also has other applications.

Construct Validity. The degree to which an instrument measures the theoretical construct or trait that it was designed to measure (e.g., severity adjustment scales are tools for measuring staffing needs).

Content Validity. The degree to which the instrument adequately represents the universe of content; includes judgments by experts or respondents about the degree to which the test appears to measure the relevant construct.

Continuous. Uninterrupted extension in sequence or an uninterrupted flow.

Control Chart. Used to statistically illustrate upper and lower limits of a process and the variation of an organization's process within those limits.

Convenience Sampling. Approach allows the use of any available group of subjects. For example, may include all patients at an organization who are undergoing a certain procedure over a 12-month period.

Corrective Action Plan (CAP). Also known as plan of correction, improvement plan, and action plan. Describes documents that organize improvements needed for organizations to be in full compliance with standards or regulations. These plans often are written in response to a survey, inspection, or gap analyses from assessments that define observations as well as recommendations for actions to achieve compliance for a given standard.

Cost-Benefit Analysis (CBA). Performed for capital expenditure requests to determine the viability and broader benefits of such expenditures. This tool helps organizations better utilize financial and human resources and includes a time frame that demonstrates the costs and benefits of the project over specific periods of time.

Criterion-Related Validity. The extent that the score on the instrument can be related to a criterion (the behavior that the instrument is supposed to predict). Can be either predictive or concurrent.

Cultural Screen. A change management tool focusing on the cultural aspect of change and identifying those factors associated with the culture of the organization that should be assessed to achieve successful change.

Culture. The set of shared attitudes, values, goals, and practices that characterizes a company or corporation. A system of beliefs and actions that characterize a particular group. Culture also refers to norms of behavior and shared values among a group of people. The social "glue" that holds people together. At the heart of culture is the notion of shared values (what is important) and behavioral "norms" (the way things are done). Cultures are described as strong when the core values are intensely held and widely shared.

Customer. The person or entity that receives the process, product, or service and therefore defines the quality of products or services received. Customer focus is a value central to any improvement initiative.

Dashboards. Used to represent key management and performance indicators. Can be used as a data-mining tool to synchronize and synthesize vast amounts of data into visual representations. Can be used for analyzing and forecasting various organizational systems.

Data. The abstract representation of things, facts, concepts, and instructions that are stored in a defined format and structure on a passive medium (e.g., paper, computer, microfilm).

Decision Support System. Deals with functions including strategic planning and marketing; resource allocation; performance evaluation and monitoring; product evaluation and services; and medical management (e.g., evidence-based practice, clinical pathways).

Delphi Method. Combination of brainstorming, multivoting, and nominal group techniques. This technique is utilized when group members are not in one location, and frequently is conducted by mail and or e-mail when a meeting is not feasible.

Deployment Chart. Used to project schedules for complex tasks and their associated subtasks. It usually is used with a task for which the time for completion is known; used to determine who has responsibility for the parts of a plan or project. Also called a planning grid.

Diffusion. The process by which an innovation or new idea is communicated through certain channels over time among members of a social system (dissemination can be synonymous with diffusion).

Do. Make changes on an experimental, pilot basis.

Effective. Care provided based on scientific knowledge as to who will likely benefit, and restrain from providing care when it is not likely to benefit the patient (Institute of Medicine [IOM] Six Aims).

Efficient. Care provided in ways that avoid waste, including waste of equipment, supplies, ideas, and energy (IOM Six Aims).

Empowerment. The giving away of power traditionally held by the manager. It typically involves a higher level of information sharing, decision making, and problem solving at the level closest to the situation, and shared recognition.

Equitable. Care does not vary in quality because of patients' personal characteristics such as gender, ethnicity, geographic location, and socioeconomic status (IOM Six Aims).

Evidence-Based Medicine. The conscientious, explicit, and judicious use of current best evidence in making decisions about the care of individual patients.

Expectancy Theory. Is concerned with how individuals decide which behaviors to engage in and how much effort they should give to that behavior; focuses on the individual's perception of effort-to-performance and performance-to-outcomes links.

Expert Sampling. Type of purposive sampling that involves selecting experts in a given area because of their access to the information relevant to the study.

Fail Forward. Approach whereby one faces failure rather than avoids failure.

Failure Mode and Effects Analysis (FMEA). A preventive approach to identify failures and opportunities for error; can be used for processes as well as equipment. An FMEA is a systematic method of identifying and preventing failures before they occur.

First-Order Change. Comprises small, relatively easy steps; requires minimal effort to achieve; rarely has a significant effect on complex systems or organizations.

Fitness for Use. As explained in The Juran Triology, the cost of quality accounting means that there is a break-even point of less than 100%. Beyond a certain point, the cost of providing quality exceeds the value of the incremental improvement in quality.

Flowchart/Process Flowchart. Graphical display of a process outlining the sequence and relationship of the pieces of the process.

Focused/Intensive Review. Those activities whereby processes or outcomes are utilizing preestablished criteria or indicators.

Force Field Analysis. A method to systematically identify the various forces that facilitate or increase the likelihood of success, and the opposite factors, those that decrease or restrain the likelihood of success or improvement in the process.

Goal. Broad, general statement specifying a purpose or desired outcome and may be more abstract in nature than an objective (one goal can have several objectives). Establishing a goal is the initial step in the strategic planning process and sets the direction for the activities to follow.

Green Belt. Organization member who usually carries out projects. This individual is knowledgeable about Six Sigma methods but has received less training.

Guiding Principles. The organization's attitudes and policies for employees that help to direct the vision.

Healthcare Facilities Accreditation Program (HFAP). American Osteopathic Association's HFAP accredits acute-care hospitals, hospital laboratories, ambulatory care/surgery, mental health, substance abuse, and physical rehabilitation medicine facilities.

Heroes. Company role models whose ideals, character, and support of the organizational culture highlight the values and norms a company wishes to reinforce. Heroes provide a role model for success.

Histogram. Used to illustrate the variability or distribution of data; tool presents the measurement scale of values along its *x*-axis (broken into equal-sized intervals) and the frequency scale (as counts or percents) along the *y*-axis.

Hoshin Planning. A Japanese term that means policy deployment; Hoshin planning is a component of the total quality management/quality improvement (TQM/QI) system used to ensure that the vision set forth by top management is being translated into planning objectives. Also includes the actions that both management and employees will take to accomplish long-term organizational strategic goals.

Information. Obtained when data are translated into results and statements that are useful for decision making. To be meaningful, data must be considered within the context of how they were obtained and how they are to be used.

Innovation. An idea, practice, or object that is perceived as new by those who adopt it.

Instruments. Devices that healthcare quality professionals and researchers use to obtain and record the data received from the subjects (e.g., questionnaires, rating scales, and interview transcripts).

Interrater Reliability. The degree to which two raters, operating independently, assign the same ratings in the context of observational research or in coding qualitative materials.

Interrelationship Diagram. Organizes numerous complex problems, issues, or ideas by sorting and displaying their interrelations. Requires multidirectional thinking when there is not a straight-line, cause-and-effect relationship.

Interval Data. The distance between each data point is equal (e.g., the values on a Fahrenheit thermometer).

Joint Commission on Accreditation of Healthcare Organizations (JCAHO). Accreditation commission that aims to improve the safety of care using accreditation and certification as risk-reduction activities; compliance with standards is intended to reduce the risk of adverse outcomes.

Knowledge Management. The process of collecting information about the spread with the measurement and feedback component for modifying the spread process as necessary; focuses on the knowledge that people need to do their work, improve services, remain current with changing needs, and develop innovative solutions.

Leadership. The ability to influence an individual or group toward achievement of goals.

Lean Enterprise. Includes the application of value stream analysis, a tool for exposing waste, and root cause analysis, which is a method for pursuing perfection. Lean enterprise also includes the use of new technologies to facilitate more efficient practices. Major focus in a lean enterprise is to eliminate waste in the following areas: production, waiting time, inappropriate processing, inventory, transporting, and defects.

Management Information System (MIS). Can contain both the manual and the automated methods to provide information for decision making. Other names for an MIS, which are used interchangeably, include data-processing structure, clinical information system, medical information system, hospital information system, or decision support system.

Matrix Diagram. Displays the connection between each idea or issue in one group to one or more groups. Can show the relationship between two items as well as the strength of the relationship.

Mean. The sum of all scores or values divided by the total number of scores. The mean, also known as the average, is the most widely used measure of central tendency in statistical tests of significance.

Median. The measure of central tendency that corresponds to the middle score; that is, the point on a numerical scale above which and below which 50 percent of the cases fall.

Mission. Refers to the organization's purpose or reason for existing. It basically answers questions such as, "Why are we here?" "Whom do we serve?" and "What do we do?"

Misuse. When patients receive appropriate medical services that are provided poorly, exposing them to added risk of preventable complications.

Mode. The score or value that occurs most frequently in a distribution of scores. Of the three measures of central tendency, the mode is the easiest to determine; simply determine which value occurs most often in the data set.

Multiple Regression Analysis. Estimates the effects of two or more independent variables (x) on a dependent measure (y).

Multivoting. An easy, quick method for determining the most popular or important items from a list. This method utilizes a series of votes to cut the list in half each time, thus reducing the number of items to be considered.

National Committee for Quality Assurance (NCQA). Accreditation committee that evaluates the quality of care and service provided by healthcare organizations. NCQA assesses organization performance against standards for care and service delivery, including the Health Plan Employer Data and Information Set (HEDIS).

Nominal Data. Called count, discrete, or qualitative data. In statistical process control, these are known as attributes data. Binary data are categorical data with only two possibilities (e.g., gender).

Nominal Group Technique. A group decision-making process for generating a large number of ideas in which each member works by himself or herself.

Nonparametric Tests. Statistical tests used with categorical (attributes) data and should be used with ordinal data, especially if the ordinal categories have a small range of possible values or a nonnormal distribution.

Norms of Behavior. Common or pervasive ways of acting that are found in a group.

Objectives. Specific statements that detail how the goals will be achieved; they therefore are relatively narrow and concrete. Objectives represent the organization's commitment to achieving specific outcomes.

Observability/Visibility. The degree to which the use of an innovation and the results it produces are visible to those who should consider it.

Ordinal Data. Characteristics are put into categories and are rank-ordered. Assignment to the categories is not arbitrary. Examples of ordinal scale data are nursing staff rank (nurse level 1, nurse level 2), education (BS, MS, MD), or attitude toward research scale (strong agree, agree, neutral, disagree, strongly disagree).

Organizational Learning. Describes organizations skilled at creating, acquiring and transferring knowledge, and at modifying behavior to reflect new knowledge and insights.

Outcomes. The results of care processes (e.g., how patients fare as a result of treatment, satisfaction, length, and quality of life).

Overuse. When patients undergo treatment or procedures from which they do not benefit (e.g., 50% of X rays in back pain patients are unnecessary).

Parametric Tests. Statistical tests used with data measured on a continuous scale (i.e., interval or ratio data, which are also known as variables data).

Pareto Diagram/Pareto Chart. Tool used to prioritize a series of problems or possible causes of problems. Displays a series of bars in which the priority for problem solving can easily be seen by the varying height of the bars.

Patient-Centered. Care that is respectful and responsive to patient preferences, needs, and values. Further, patient values should guide all clinical decisions (IOM Six Aims).

Patient Safety. Any improvement effort focused on eliminating medical errors; the degree to which the healthcare environment is free from hazards or dangers.

Pay for Performance. Incentives that drive breakthrough performance to improve the quality of care and service rendered by healthcare providers. Typically includes performance metrics, public report cards, and payment differential for providing better quality care and service.

Performance Management. The use of performance management information to effect positive change in organizational culture, systems and processes, by helping to set agreed-upon performance goals, allocating and prioritizing resources, informing managers to either confirm or change current policy or program direction to meet those goals, and sharing results of performance in pursuing those goals.

Performance Monitoring. Monitoring the impact and effectiveness of the quality improvement action and collecting additional data.

Plan. Question the capacity or capability of a process. Pose theories on how to improve the process and predict measurable outcomes.

Plan, Do, Check, Act (PDCA). Four-step process designed to continuously improve quality, originally conceived by Shewhart.

Plan, Do, Study, Act (PDSA). Later adaptation by Deming of the PDCA cycle; also is referred to as the Deming Cycle, or the Deming Wheel.

Population (*N*). The total aggregate or group (e.g., all cases that meet a designated set of criteria for practitioners, all patients who have died at a particular hospital, or all registered nurses with a tenure of 10 years or more).

Prioritization Matrix. Organizes tasks, issues, or actions and prioritizes them based on agreed-upon criteria. The tool combines the tree diagram and the L-shaped matrix diagram, displaying the best possible effect.

Probability Sampling. Sampling that requires every element in the population to have an equal or random chance of being selected for inclusion in the sample.

Procedural Justice. Focuses on fairness with respect to processes or procedures used to allocate outcomes.

Process. Involved with how the care is delivered (how patients were diagnosed and treated; the activities involved in prevention, diagnosis, and treatment).

Process Analysis. A method of analyzing data using industrial quality improvement techniques to improve clinical or administrative outcomes. Process analysis occurs whenever a group of individuals diagrams a healthcare process.

Process Decision Program Chart. Maps out the identified events and contingencies that can occur from a problem statement to its solution. Attempts to identify potential deviations from the desired process, thus allowing the team to anticipate and prevent the deviation.

Purposive/Judgment Sampling. Method selects a particular group or groups based on certain criteria. Subjective, because the researcher uses his or her judgment to decide who is representative of the population.

Quality Circle (QC). A group of employees who perform similar duties and meet on a regular basis, with or without management, to discuss quality and productivity problems and propose solutions and/or suggestions for improvement.

Quality Control. Evaluation of actual quality performance, comparing actual performance to quality goals and acting on the differences.

Quality Improvement. Means by which quality performance is achieved at unprecedented levels by establishing the infrastructure needed to secure annual quality improvement; identifying the specific areas for improvement; establishing clear accountability for bringing QI projects to a successful conclusion; and providing the resources, motivation, and training needed by the teams (i.e., diagnose the causes, stimulate establishment of a remedy, and establish controls to hold the gains).

Quality Improvement Teams. Can be *natural work teams,* for example, teams with members who work "permanently" as a team each day to complete the task; can be *cross-functional,* as with an operating-room team; or *intact,* such as a team of nurses in a particular unit.

Quality Planning. The activity of developing the products and processes required to meet customer needs by determining who the customers are as well as their needs; developing product features and processes that respond to needs and produce desired product features; and transferring the resulting plans to the operating forces.

Quota Sampling. Researcher makes a judgment decision about the best type of sample for the investigation and prespecifies characteristics of the sample to increase its representativeness.

Range. The difference between the highest and lowest values in a distribution of scores.

Rapid Cycle Improvement. Strategy whereby organizations collaborate to identify and prioritize aims for improvement, and gain access to methods, tools, and materials that will enable them to conduct sophisticated, evidence-based quality improvement activities that they could not conduct individually.

Ratio Data. The distance between each point is equal and there is a true zero (e.g., weight and height).

Readiness. Being prepared mentally or physically for some experience or action, immediately available, or ready for immediate use.

Reengineering. Efforts focused on work force redesign; restructuring systems and departments into more efficient processes.

Regression Analysis. Based on statistical correlations or associations among variables.

Relative Advantage. The degree to which an innovation is perceived as better than the idea it supersedes.

Reliability. The extent to which an experiment, test, or measuring procedure yields the same results on repeated trials.

Resilience. The process of adapting well in the face of adversity, trauma, tragedy, threats, or even significant sources of stress—such as family and relationship problems, serious health problems, or workplace and financial stressors.

Reversibility. The ability to stop the adoption or use of the innovation and return to a normal or "safe" position if the innovation is not effective.

Risk Adjustment. Technique used to take into account or to control the fact that different patients with the same diagnosis might have additional conditions or characteristics that could affect how well they respond to treatment.

Risk Management. Strategies deployed to protect the organization from financial losses, which may arise because of the risks to which it is exposed.

Run/Trend Chart. Graphic displays of data points over time. Run charts are control charts without the control limits.

Safe. Avoid injuries to patients from care that is intended to help them (IOM Six Aims).

Sample. Selection of cases from the accessible population to provide a logical way of making statements about a larger group based on a smaller group and to permit researchers to make inferences or generalize from the sample to the population.

Scatter Diagram. Tool used to display possible cause and effect. Can determine the extent to which two variables (quality effects or process causes) relate to one another. Often used in combination with fishbone or Pareto diagrams/charts.

Second-Order Change. Complex and requires a significant change in behavior to achieve desired new ways of performing or new processes.

Severity of Harm. An estimation of how serious the effects or harm would be if a given failure did occur.

Shared Values. Important concerns and goals shared by most of the people in a group; they tend to shape group behavior and often persist over time even when group membership changes.

Simple Process. Allows people to follow a prescribed procedure to get the same results every time; for example, cooking with a recipe that has been tested ensures replicability without particular expertise (e.g., running preprogrammed or automated reports).

Simple Random Sampling. Each individual in the sampling frame (all subjects in the population) has an equal chance of being chosen (e.g., pulling a name out of a hat containing all possible names).

Simplicity/Complexity. The degree to which an innovation is perceived as simple to understand and use.

Six Sigma. A rigorous methodology that uses data and statistical analysis to measure and improve performance. Quality is improved by eliminating errors in production and service-related processes. Six Sigma is based on the concept of the normal distribution or curve and the belief that there is a point, six standard deviations from the mean, where there should be almost zero defects. Therefore, error rates should not exceed 3.4 defects per million opportunities (dpmo).

Snowball Sampling. A subtype of convenience sampling that involves subjects suggesting other subjects for inclusion in the study, so that the sampling process gains momentum. This type of sampling process gains subjects who are difficult to identify, but are known to others because of an informal network.

Special-Cause. In statistical process control, it describes problems that stem from isolated occurrences that are outside the system.

Special-Cause Variation. Occurs when an activity falls outside the control limits or there is an obvious nonrandom pattern around the central line. This type of variation should be interpreted as a trend and investigated.

Standard Deviation. An average of the deviations from the mean, it is the most frequently used statistic for measuring the degree of variability in a set of scores. Standard refers to the fact that the deviation indicates a group's average spread of scores or values around their mean; deviation indicates how much each score is scattered from the mean.

Statistical Process Control (SPC). Allows management to determine a range of random variation that always occurs in a process. SPC describes two types of causes of random variation: common cause and special cause.

Strategic Goal. Broadly stated or long-term outcome written as an overall statement that relates to a philosophy, a purpose, or a desired outcome.

Strategic Objective. Specific statements that are written in measurable and observable terms using quantitative and qualitative measurement criteria. Written as an action-oriented statement, it indicates the minimum acceptable level of performance and specific time limit or degree of accuracy.

Strategic Planning. The development and codification of a major direction for an organization's future.

Strategy. The plans and activities developed by an organization in pursuit of its goals and objectives, particularly in regard to positioning itself to meet external demands relative to its competition.

Stratification. Breaks down single numbers into meaningful categories or classification to focus corrective action; used to isolate and illuminate improvement opportunities.

Stratification Chart. Designed to show where a problem does and does not occur, or to demonstrate underlying patterns.

Stratified Random Sampling. A subpopulation is a stratum, and strata are two or more homogeneous subpopulations. After the population has been divided into strata, each member of a stratum has an equal probability of being selected (e.g., sex, ethnicity, patients with particular diseases, or patients living in certain parts of the country).

Structure. The resources available for care delivery (e.g., the qualifications of practitioners and facilities/technology available to them).

Symbols. Things that represent an idea. The purpose of symbols is to reflect the culture, trigger values and norms, and help people make sense of their organization.

System. Regularly interacting or interdependent group of items forming a unified whole; a framework for seeing interrelationships, rather than things; for seeing patterns of change rather than static "snapshots."

Systematic Sampling. After randomly selecting the first case, this method involves drawing every *n*-th element from a population (e.g., picking every third name from a list of possible names).

Team. A group of people who are interdependent with respect to information, resources, and skills and who seek to combine their efforts to achieve a common goal.

Timely. Wait times and harmful delays for those who receive and provide care should be eliminated (IOM Six Aims).

Total Quality. Best defined as an attitude, an orientation that permeates an entire organization, and the way that an organization performs its internal and external business. Total quality integrates fundamental management techniques, existing improvement efforts, and the use of technical tools utilizing a disciplined statistical quality control (SQC).

Total Quality Management (TQM). An approach to organizational development and change that ensures the organization meets or exeeds customer expectations; a strategic, integrated management system that involves all managers and employees and uses quantitative methods to continuously improve an organization's processes to meet and exceed customer needs, wants, and expectations.

Tree Diagram. Maps out the full range of paths and tasks that are involved in the process and must be accomplished in order to achieve a goal; resembles an organizational chart.

Trialability. The degree to which an innovation can be tested on a small scale.

***t* Test.** Used to analyze the difference between two means to determine whether the difference between two group means is significant; a distinction must be made regarding the two groups.

Uncertainty. The fear and discomfort associated with the implementation of the innovation.

Underuse. When patients do not receive beneficial health services (e.g., 50% of heart attack victims fail to receive beta-blockers).

Unfreezing. Beliefs, expectations, and norms that can be remolded into new beliefs and behaviors. Through a process of learning new information, attitudes, and processes, people are able to redefine their current beliefs and "refreeze" these new concepts into their behaviors.

Utilization Management. An organized, comprehensive approach to analyze, direct, and conserve organizational resources, so as to provide care that is both high in quality and cost-effective (e.g., medical necessity appropriateness review; discharge planning and monitoring; overutilization and underutilization surveillance; and identification of over, and underutilization).

Utilization Review Accreditation Commission (URAC). Accreditation organization for case management, claims processing, consumer-directed healthcare, core accreditation, credentials verification organization, disease management, health call center, health network, health plan, health provider credentialing, health utilization management, health Web site, Health Insurance Portability and Accountability Act (HIPAA) privacy, HIPAA security, independent review, and workers' compensation utilization management.

Validity. The degree to which an instrument measures what it is intended to measure. Validity usually is more difficult to establish than reliability.

Values. The beliefs and philosophy within an organization that establish the basis for the operation and provide guidelines for daily behavior.

Variability. The degree to which values on a set of scores differ.

Variation Analysis. Used to explain statistically significant differences in the data. These differences may be due to clinical factors, patient characteristics, data collection (e.g., sampling characteristics), or organizational characteristics (e.g., staffing).

Vision. An organization's statement of its goals for the future, described in measurable terms that clarify the direction for everyone in the organization. An organization's direction is built upon its mission and is guided, through leadership, by its vision.

Work Motivation. The psychological forces that determine the *direction* of a person's behavior in an organization, a person's level of *effort*, and a person's level of *persistence.*

Index

Note: A page number with an italic f indicates that entry is included in a figure; a page number with an italic t indicates that entry is included in a table.

D

E

F

J

K

L

M

N

O

S

T

KEY CODE

BVwvYICgtz

Q SOLUTIONS

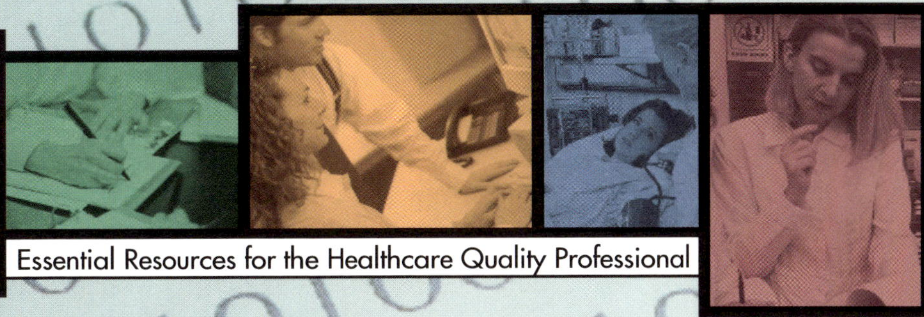

Thank you for purchasing *Q Solutions: Essential Resources for the Healthcare Quality Professional*! You now have access to the Q Solutions Web site:

Step 1: Go to www.q-solutions.org

Step 2: Log in with

- Your unique key: (insert key code listed above)
- Password: you will need to set this up on your first visit to the Web site.

Please note that you will need to provide NAHQ with some brief information when you log in for the first time. Keep this information handy as you will need it to access the site.

Any questions? Please contact NAHQ's member services department at 800/966-9392 or info@nahq.org

NAHQ
National Association for Healthcare Quality

Login name: ______________________________

Password: ______________________________